INSULIN RESISTANCE DIET COOKBOOK FOR BEGINNERS

A Comprehensive Guide to Lower Blood Sugar and Regain Your Health

By

Hector Wiggins

Table of Contents

INTRODUCTION

In the heart of bustling city life, where the rhythm of each day often dictates our choices, a whisper emerged—a whisper that held the power to rewrite the narrative of health for beginners. Picture, if you will, the bustling streets where lives unfold, where people navigate the complexities of modern living. Among them, there is you—a beginner seeking a path to conquer insulin resistance and embrace a life brimming with vitality.

As the sun sets on a day filled with both triumphs and challenges, you find yourself at the crossroads of choice. The echo of a diagnosis, perhaps recent or long-standing, reverberates—a challenge named insulin resistance. But within every challenge, there lies an opportunity, a story waiting to unfold, a journey yet to be embarked upon.

Our story begins not with deprivation or
restrictive measures but with the promise of
culinary exploration—a journey that transcends
the notion of a mere cookbook. This is an
odyssey designed for beginners, where the
kitchen becomes a realm of empowerment,
and each meal a brushstroke on the canvas of
your well-being.

Imagine opening the pages of this cookbook
and stepping into a world where flavors dance,
and nutrients play the role of silent healers.
Each recipe, a testament to the balance sought
in the face of insulin resistance, is a melody
composed for your health, a harmony created
for your journey.

Let me share with you the tale of Michel, a beginner like yourself, who, armed with this very cookbook, transformed her kitchen into a sanctuary of well-being. As she flipped through the pages, she discovered the art of crafting balanced meals that not only satisfied her taste buds but also nurtured her body, inching her closer to triumph over insulin resistance.

Michel's story is just one thread in the rich tapestry of this cookbook, woven with the principles of the insulin resistance diet. It's a tale of understanding, empowerment, and the joy that emanates from reclaiming control over your health.

So, dear reader, as you embark on this culinary expedition, let the aroma of wholesome ingredients guide you. Allow the sizzle in the pan to be a promise—a promise of embracing a lifestyle where each meal is a step towards defeating insulin resistance.

This cookbook is more than recipes; it's an invitation to a transformative journey where you, the beginner, become the hero of your own story.

Turn the page, and let the adventure begin. Welcome to the "Insulin Resistance Diet Cookbook for Beginners," where each recipe is a step towards your triumph, and every meal is a celebration of your well-being.

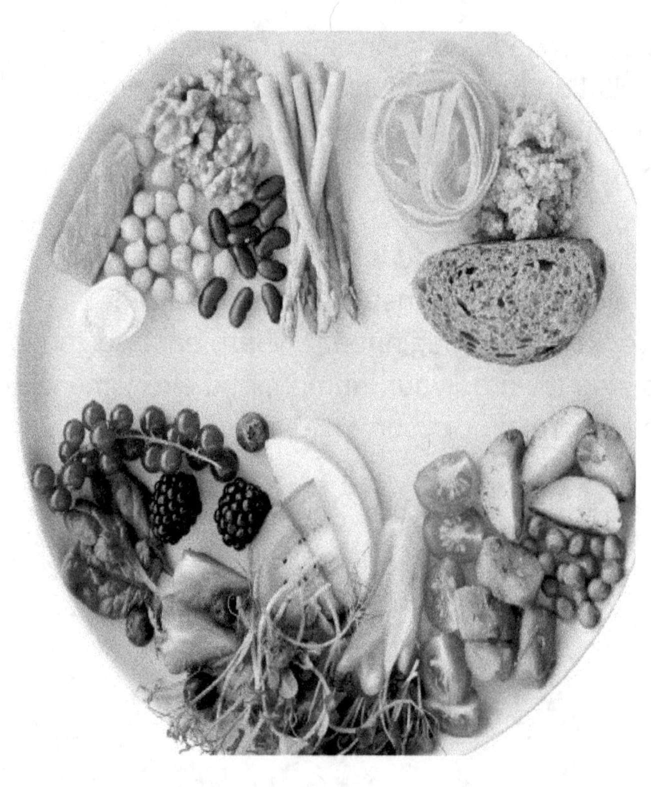

Understanding Insulin Resistance

 Insulin resistance is a complex physiological condition that involves the body's response to insulin, a vital hormone secreted by the pancreas. To comprehend insulin resistance, we must first delve into the intricate dance between insulin, glucose, and the body's cells.

Insulin's Role:
Insulin acts as a key that unlocks cells, allowing glucose (sugar) to enter. This process is crucial for energy production and regulation of blood sugar levels.

Glucose Uptake: Our digestive system converts food, particularly carbohydrates, into glucose when we eat it. Insulin helps cells absorb glucose so they can use it as fuel.

The Cellular Disconnect:
In individuals with insulin resistance, cells become less responsive to the signals of insulin. Despite the pancreas releasing more insulin to compensate, cells resist its efforts, leading to elevated blood sugar levels.

Consequences of Insulin Resistance:
High levels of circulating glucose can contribute to various health issues. It may lead to the development of type 2 diabetes, cardiovascular problems, and other metabolic disturbances.

Causes and Risk Factors:
Insulin resistance can stem from a combination of genetic and lifestyle factors. Sedentary habits, poor dietary choices, obesity, and a family history of diabetes are common contributors.

Recognizing Signs and Symptoms:
Insulin resistance often manifests subtly.
Symptoms may include fatigue, increased
hunger, and difficulty losing weight. However,
the condition can progress without noticeable
signs.

Diagnostic Measures:
Medical professionals use various tests, such
as fasting blood sugar and insulin levels, as
well as the HbA1c test, to diagnose insulin
resistance. These assessments provide insight
into how effectively the body manages blood
sugar over time.

Lifestyle Management:
Lifestyle modifications, including dietary
changes, regular physical activity, and weight
management, play pivotal roles in addressing
insulin resistance. A balanced diet and an
active lifestyle can enhance insulin sensitivity,
helping the body respond more effectively to
insulin's signals.

Definition of Insulin Resistance

A metabolic disorder known as insulin resistance occurs when the body's cells lose their sensitivity to the pancreatic hormone insulin. Insulin is a key player in blood sugar regulation because it makes it easier for cells to absorb glucose and use it as fuel. When a person has insulin resistance, their cells do not respond to insulin as well, which raises blood glucose levels.

Insulin binds to cell surface receptors in a physiologically normal mechanism that instructs cells to absorb glucose. Nevertheless, this signaling pathway is compromised in insulin resistance. The pancreas tries to overcome the resistance and maintain normal blood sugar levels by producing more insulin in response. Blood sugar levels may grow over time if the body is unable to produce enough insulin to offset resistance, which may result in health problems including type 2 diabetes.

Numerous factors, including heredity, obesity, sedentary lifestyles, and dietary choices, are frequently linked to insulin resistance. A balanced diet, frequent exercise, and weight control are common lifestyle changes used to address insulin resistance in order to improve insulin sensitivity and advance metabolic health in general. For long-term wellbeing and to avoid consequences from high blood sugar, it is essential to recognize and treat insulin resistance.

The Impact of Insulin on Blood Sugar and Health

Insulin, often referred to as the body's metabolic maestro, plays a pivotal role in orchestrating the delicate balance of blood sugar and overall health. Its impact is multifaceted, influencing various physiological processes that contribute to the body's well-being.

Insulin is the primary hormone that controls blood sugar levels. Glucose is produced by the digestive system from the chemicals we eat, particularly carbs. Insulin serves as a gatekeeper, permitting glucose to enter cells where it is converted into energy.

Cellular Energy Production:
Inside cells, glucose is converted into energy through a process known as cellular respiration. Insulin ensures that cells receive an adequate supply of glucose, enabling them to function optimally.

Storage of Excess Glucose:
Insulin plays a crucial role in storing excess glucose for future energy needs. It facilitates the conversion of surplus glucose into glycogen in the liver and muscles, acting as a reservoir for times when blood sugar levels decrease.

Prevention of Hyperglycemia:
By promoting the uptake of glucose into cells, insulin prevents the accumulation of excess sugar in the bloodstream. This is essential for preventing hyperglycemia, which can lead to various health complications.

Protein and Fat Metabolism:
Insulin influences the metabolism of proteins
and fats. It facilitates the synthesis of proteins
and helps in storing excess dietary fat,
contributing to overall metabolic balance.

Inhibition of Gluconeogenesis:
Insulin inhibits gluconeogenesis, a process
where the liver produces glucose from
non-carbohydrate sources. This inhibition helps
maintain stable blood sugar levels.

Cell Growth and Repair:
Beyond its role in glucose regulation, insulin
supports cell growth, repair, and maintenance.
It has anabolic effects, promoting the synthesis
of essential molecules for cellular health.

The impact of insulin on blood sugar and health is interconnected with the body's ability to maintain metabolic harmony. When this hormonal symphony functions optimally, blood sugar levels remain within a healthy range, supporting energy production, cellular function, and overall well-being. However, disruptions in insulin function, such as in insulin resistance, can lead to imbalances, emphasizing the importance of understanding and supporting insulin's crucial role in maintaining health.

Importance of Dietary Management

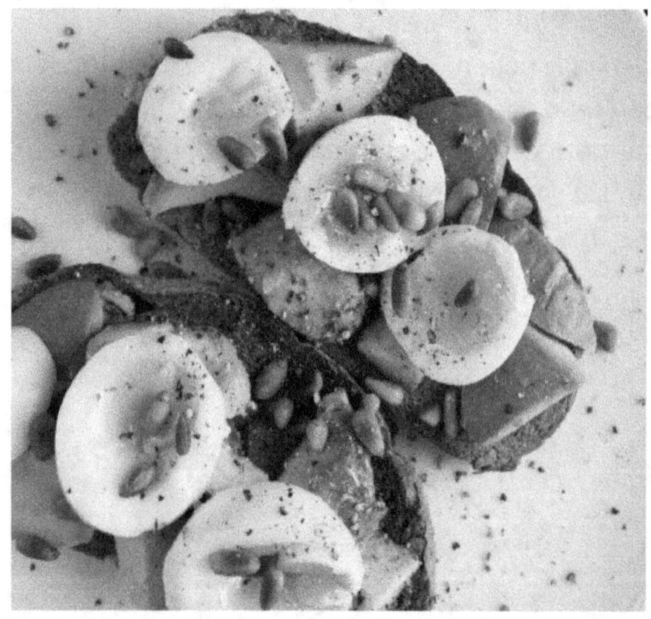

The most effective way to fight insulin resistance is through dietary management, which has a profound influence on how the body responds to insulin and regulates blood sugar. This is why it's so important:

Blood Sugar Control:
Dietary choices directly impact blood sugar levels. Managing the types and amounts of carbohydrates, particularly those with a low glycemic index, helps prevent rapid spikes in blood sugar and supports insulin sensitivity.

Balanced Macronutrients:
A well-balanced diet ensures an appropriate distribution of macronutrients—carbohydrates, proteins, and fats. This balance contributes to sustained energy, preventing excessive glucose influx and promoting overall metabolic health.

Healthy Carbohydrate Options: Opting for complex carbohydrates rather than processed foods and refined sugars promotes a gradual release of glucose and reduces the risk of sudden spikes in blood sugar. Vegetables, lentils, and whole grains are great options.

Lean Proteins:
Including lean protein sources in the diet supports muscle health and can contribute to a feeling of fullness, potentially preventing overconsumption of carbohydrates.

Essential Fats:
Incorporating healthy fats, such as those found in avocados, nuts, and olive oil, helps regulate insulin sensitivity. These fats contribute to a balanced diet without causing spikes in blood sugar.

Portion Control:
Managing portion sizes helps control calorie intake, contributing to weight management. Maintaining a healthy weight is crucial for reducing insulin resistance and improving overall metabolic function.

Fiber-Rich Foods:
Dietary fiber plays a key role in slowing down the absorption of glucose and promoting a feeling of fullness. Whole fruits, vegetables, and whole grains are excellent sources of fiber.

Limiting Processed Foods:
Processed foods often contain added sugars and unhealthy fats, contributing to insulin resistance. Limiting their consumption supports overall health and insulin sensitivity.

Regular Meal Timing:
Consistent meal timing helps regulate blood sugar levels by providing a steady supply of nutrients. Skipping meals or prolonged periods without food can lead to fluctuations in blood sugar.

Individualized Approaches:
Recognizing that dietary needs vary among individuals, an individualized approach to dietary management is crucial. Tailoring dietary plans to personal preferences, cultural considerations, and nutritional requirements enhances adherence and success.

CHAPTER ONE

Embarking on the Insulin Resistance Journey

Embarking on the insulin resistance journey is a transformative step towards understanding, managing, and reclaiming control over one's metabolic health. As you stand at the threshold of this voyage, envision it not merely as a challenge but as an opportunity for profound positive change.

Assessing Your Insulin Sensitivity:
Begin your journey by understanding your current insulin sensitivity. This involves recognizing how well your body responds to insulin's signals. Medical professionals often use tests like fasting blood sugar, insulin levels, and HbA1c to gauge this sensitivity.

Setting Personal Health Goals:
Define your health goals clearly. Whether it's achieving stable blood sugar levels, losing weight, or improving overall well-being, having specific, measurable goals provides direction and motivation for your journey.

Embracing a Lifestyle Change:
Recognize that managing insulin resistance requires lifestyle modifications. These changes encompass dietary adjustments, regular physical activity, stress management, and other wellness practices. Embrace these changes as positive investments in your health.

Understanding the Role of Nutrition:
Delve into the impact of nutrition on insulin sensitivity. Learn about the types of carbohydrates, the significance of balanced meals, and the role of macronutrients in promoting metabolic health. Consider consulting with a nutrition professional to tailor a dietary plan to your unique needs.

Exploring Physical Activity:
Physical activity is a powerful ally in managing insulin resistance. Engage in exercises that you enjoy, making them a sustainable part of your routine. Whether it's walking, cycling, or yoga, find activities that bring joy and contribute to improved insulin sensitivity.

Cultivating Stress Management Techniques:
Acknowledge the intricate connection between stress and insulin resistance. Explore stress-reducing techniques such as mindfulness, meditation, or deep breathing exercises. Cultivating a calm mindset supports your body's ability to regulate blood sugar.

Building a Support System:
Share your journey with friends, family, or support groups. A robust support system provides encouragement, accountability, and a shared understanding of the challenges and triumphs along the way.

Every step you take on the path to insulin resistance teaches you something new. Take lessons from your experiences, both the good and the bad. Recognize that although the journey may be convoluted, every lesson advances your growing comprehension of wellness.

Honoring Minor Victories: Congratulate yourself on any accomplishment, no matter how minor. Acknowledging your accomplishments, whether it's reaching a physical goal or making nutrient-rich food choices consistently, helps you stay motivated and maintain a positive outlook on your path.

Nurturing a Growth Mindset:
Approach the insulin resistance journey with a growth mindset. View challenges as opportunities to learn and grow. Embrace the journey as a continual process of self-discovery and improvement.

Remember, embarking on the insulin resistance journey is not a solitary endeavor. It's a shared exploration of well-being and resilience. As you take these initial steps, envision a future where you are not merely managing insulin resistance but thriving in a state of empowered wellness. This journey is yours to craft, and with each stride, you move closer to a life enriched by health, vitality, and self-discovery.

Assessing Your Insulin Sensitivity

Assessing insulin sensitivity is a crucial step in understanding how effectively your body responds to insulin, the hormone responsible for regulating blood sugar levels. This assessment provides valuable insights into your metabolic health and sets the stage for informed decisions on managing insulin resistance. Here's a closer look at the process:

Fasting Blood Sugar Levels:
One fundamental measure is assessing fasting blood sugar levels. This involves measuring your blood sugar after an overnight fast. Elevated fasting blood sugar may indicate reduced insulin sensitivity.

Insulin Levels:
Testing insulin levels alongside fasting blood sugar offers a more comprehensive view. Higher insulin levels in relation to blood sugar may suggest the need for closer scrutiny of insulin sensitivity.

The HbA1c test gives a quick overview of the average blood sugar levels during the previous two to three months. It provides a more comprehensive view of insulin sensitivity and blood sugar regulation by measuring glycated hemoglobin.

Oral Glucose Tolerance Test (OGTT):
An OGTT involves consuming a glucose solution, and blood sugar levels are monitored over time. This dynamic test provides a detailed assessment of how your body processes glucose and responds to insulin.

Home Glucose Monitoring:
Regular monitoring of blood sugar levels at home using a glucose meter is an empowering approach. It allows you to observe how your body reacts to different foods and lifestyle factors, providing real-time insights into your insulin sensitivity.

Consultation with Healthcare Professionals:
Seeking guidance from healthcare professionals, such as an endocrinologist or a registered dietitian, is invaluable. They can interpret test results, assess your overall health, and offer personalized recommendations based on your unique circumstances.

Assessment of Lifestyle Factors:
Recognizing lifestyle factors that influence insulin sensitivity is essential. Consider factors such as physical activity, dietary habits, stress levels, and sleep patterns. Lifestyle modifications can significantly impact insulin sensitivity.

Tracking Body Composition:
Body composition, including the distribution of fat and muscle mass, can affect insulin sensitivity. Regularly monitoring and addressing changes in body composition contribute to a comprehensive understanding of metabolic health.

Genetic Considerations:
Acknowledging genetic factors that may influence insulin sensitivity provides a more holistic perspective. While genetics play a role, lifestyle choices can modulate their impact on insulin resistance.

Regular Health Check-ups:
Routine health check-ups allow for ongoing assessment of metabolic markers. Regular monitoring creates a baseline for understanding how interventions, such as dietary changes and physical activity, influence insulin sensitivity over time.

Understanding your insulin sensitivity is not a one-time event; it is an ongoing process. Regular assessments, coupled with lifestyle modifications, empower you to take an active role in managing and improving insulin sensitivity. Embrace these insights as tools for creating a personalized approach to well-being and navigating the path toward optimal metabolic health.

Setting Personal Health Goals

Establishing clear and achievable health goals is a foundational step on your journey to managing insulin resistance through dietary choices. These goals not only provide direction but also serve as powerful motivators for sustained lifestyle changes. Here's how to set personalized health goals tailored to an insulin resistance diet:

Define Clear Objectives:
Begin by articulating specific and measurable goals. Whether it's achieving stable blood sugar levels, losing weight, or improving overall well-being, clarity in your objectives lays the groundwork for success.

Consider Your Unique Needs:
Recognize that health goals should align with your individual circumstances. Factors such as age, current health status, dietary preferences, and lifestyle constraints should inform your goal-setting process.

Focus on Blood Sugar Control:
Prioritize goals related to blood sugar control. This could involve achieving and maintaining target blood sugar levels, reducing post-meal spikes, and promoting stable glucose levels throughout the day.

Weight Management Objectives:
If weight management is a goal, set realistic targets for gradual and sustainable weight loss. Even modest weight reduction can significantly improve insulin sensitivity and overall metabolic health.

Balanced Nutrition Goals:
Emphasize goals related to balanced nutrition. Consider incorporating more whole, nutrient-dense foods while reducing processed and high-sugar options. Aim for a well-rounded diet that supports overall health.

Meal Timing and Frequency:
Establish goals regarding meal timing and frequency. Consistent meal patterns, including regular, balanced meals and appropriate snacks, can help regulate blood sugar levels and enhance insulin sensitivity.

Physical Activity Targets:
Integrate physical activity into your goals. Set achievable targets for exercise frequency, duration, and type. Regular physical activity positively influences insulin sensitivity and complements dietary efforts.

Incorporate objectives pertaining to mindful eating practices. Practice portion control, become conscious of your hunger and fullness cues, and enjoy every bite. Eating with awareness promotes a positive connection with food.

Stress Management Objectives:
Acknowledge the impact of stress on insulin resistance. Set goals for incorporating stress-reducing activities, such as meditation, deep breathing exercises, or hobbies, into your routine.

Consult with Healthcare Professionals:
Engage in a collaborative goal-setting process with healthcare professionals. Consulting with a healthcare provider, registered dietitian, or diabetes educator ensures that your goals align with your health status and are safe and effective.

Monitor and Celebrate Achievements:
Create a framework for monitoring accomplishments. Keep a close eye on important metrics like weight, blood sugar levels, and physical activity accomplishments. Reward minor accomplishments along the journey to keep yourself motivated.

Adapt Goals as Needed:
Recognize that goals may need adjustment based on evolving circumstances. Be flexible in adapting your objectives to ensure they remain realistic and attainable throughout your insulin resistance journey.

By setting personalized health goals for your insulin resistance diet, you are not just outlining aspirations; you are creating a roadmap to a healthier and more resilient future. These goals serve as guiding lights, providing direction, motivation, and a tangible framework for the positive changes you are determined to make on your path to improved metabolic well-being.

Preparing for a Lifestyle Change

Embarking on a journey to manage insulin resistance through lifestyle changes requires careful preparation and a commitment to fostering sustainable habits. Here's how to effectively prepare for this transformative lifestyle change:

Educate Yourself:
Begin by acquiring knowledge about insulin resistance, its impact on health, and the role of lifestyle in its management. Understanding the principles behind the insulin resistance diet empowers you to make informed decisions.

Set Realistic Expectations:
Establish realistic expectations for the lifestyle changes you plan to implement. Recognize that meaningful progress may take time, and setting achievable goals contributes to a positive and sustainable approach.

Assess Current Lifestyle Habits:
Reflect on your current lifestyle habits, including dietary choices, physical activity levels, sleep patterns, and stress management. Identify areas for improvement and consider how these factors may contribute to insulin resistance.

Consult with Healthcare Professionals:
Seek guidance from healthcare professionals, such as a healthcare provider, registered dietitian, or diabetes educator. Their expertise ensures that your lifestyle changes align with your health status, and they can provide personalized recommendations.

Create a Support System:
Share your decision to make lifestyle changes with friends, family, or a support group. Having a support system provides encouragement, accountability, and understanding as you navigate the challenges and celebrate successes.

Plan Your Meals:
Develop a meal plan that aligns with the principles of the insulin resistance diet. This plan should include balanced meals, nutrient-dense foods, and appropriate portion sizes. Preparing meals in advance can contribute to consistency.

Stock a Diabetes-Friendly Pantry:
Ensure your kitchen is stocked with diabetes-friendly staples. This includes whole grains, lean proteins, healthy fats, and a variety of colorful vegetables. Having these ingredients readily available makes it easier to make nutritious choices.

Schedule Regular Physical Activity:
Incorporate regular physical activity into your routine. Choose activities you enjoy, and gradually increase intensity and duration over time. Aim for a mix of aerobic exercise, strength training, and flexibility exercises.

Practice Stress Management Techniques:
Integrate stress management techniques into
your daily routine. This could include
mindfulness practices, deep breathing
exercises, or engaging in activities that bring
joy and relaxation.

Establish a Sleep Routine:
Prioritize sleep as an essential component of
your lifestyle change. Establish a consistent
sleep routine, create a comfortable sleep
environment, and aim for the recommended
duration of sleep each night.

Prepare for Setbacks:
Recognize that setbacks may occur, and that's
okay. Be prepared to learn from setbacks,
adjust your approach if needed, and continue
moving forward with resilience and
determination.

Celebrate Small Wins:
Acknowledge and celebrate small victories along the way. Whether it's consistently following your meal plan, achieving a fitness milestone, or managing stress more effectively, each success is a step toward improved well-being.

By carefully preparing for a lifestyle change on the insulin resistance diet, you lay the foundations for lasting success. This approach involves a holistic commitment to not only dietary modifications but also to physical activity, stress management, and overall well-being. Through thoughtful preparation and ongoing dedication, you position yourself for a transformative journey towards better health and metabolic resilience.

CHAPTER TWO

Foundations of the Insulin Resistance Diet

The insulin resistance diet is built on a set of principles designed to manage blood sugar levels and enhance insulin sensitivity. These foundations serve as a blueprint for creating a dietary approach that supports overall health and well-being:

Maintaining a Balanced Diet: Give equal importance to the three macronutrients of proteins, lipids, and carbs. Appropriate distribution of these nutrients supports sustained energy throughout the day and aids in blood sugar regulation.

Recognizing Glycemic Index: Take into account a food's glycemic index (GI). Make an effort to include low-GI foods, which release glucose gradually and help to prevent sharp rises in blood sugar. Legumes, whole grains, and non-starchy veggies fall under this category.

Portion Control:
Practice portion control to manage caloric intake and prevent overeating. Controlling portions aids in weight management, a key factor in improving insulin sensitivity.

Choosing Complex Carbohydrates:
Opt for complex carbohydrates over refined sugars. Whole grains, vegetables, and legumes provide fiber, vitamins, and minerals while offering a gradual release of glucose, supporting stable blood sugar levels.

Including Lean Proteins:
Incorporate lean protein sources into meals.
Protein helps maintain muscle mass,
contributes to a feeling of fullness, and does
not significantly impact blood sugar levels.

Choosing Good Fats: Make smart fat choices
from foods like avocados, almonds, seeds, and
olive oil. These fats do not negatively impact
insulin sensitivity and are beneficial to general
health.

Fiber-Rich Foods: Give fruits, vegetables,
whole grains, and other foods high on the
priority list. Fiber increases satiety and aids in
blood sugar regulation by slowing down the
absorption of glucose.

Limiting Processed Foods:
Minimize the consumption of processed foods that often contain added sugars, unhealthy fats, and refined carbohydrates. Whole, minimally processed foods contribute to a nutrient-dense diet.

Regular Meal Timing:
Establish regular meal timing to provide a steady supply of nutrients throughout the day. Consistent meal patterns contribute to stable blood sugar levels and support metabolic health.

Hydration:
Stay hydrated with water as the primary beverage. Proper hydration supports overall health and can aid in appetite control.

Individualized Approach:
Recognize the importance of individualization.
Dietary needs can vary, and factors such as
age, activity level, and underlying health
conditions should inform personalized dietary
choices.

Monitoring Blood Sugar Levels:
Consider monitoring blood sugar levels
regularly, especially if recommended by
healthcare professionals. This practice
provides valuable feedback on how dietary
choices impact your metabolic response.

Consulting Healthcare Professionals:
Seek guidance from healthcare professionals,
such as a registered dietitian or healthcare
provider. Their expertise ensures that your
dietary approach aligns with your unique health
status and goals.

Insulin Resistance 101

Insulin resistance is a fundamental concept in metabolic health, shaping the landscape of conditions like type 2 diabetes and influencing overall well-being. Here's a breakdown of the essential aspects in Insulin Resistance 101:

Insulin's Role:
Insulin is a hormone produced by the pancreas. Its primary role is to facilitate the uptake of glucose (sugar) into cells, providing energy for various bodily functions.

Cellular Resistance:
In individuals with insulin resistance, cells become less responsive to the signals of insulin. This resistance hinders the efficient uptake of glucose by cells, leading to elevated levels of sugar in the bloodstream.

Compensatory Insulin Production:
To overcome resistance and maintain normal
blood sugar levels, the pancreas produces
more insulin. Initially, this compensatory
mechanism keeps blood sugar within a typical
range.

Progression Over Time:
As insulin resistance persists, the pancreas
may struggle to produce sufficient insulin to
compensate. This can result in a gradual rise in
blood sugar levels, increasing the risk of
developing type 2 diabetes.

Contributing variables: A number of
variables, such as aging, obesity, poor dietary
choices, sedentary lifestyles, and heredity, can
lead to insulin resistance. It is essential to
comprehend these elements for efficient
management.

Relationships to Health Conditions:
Abdominal obesity, elevated cholesterol, high blood pressure, and metabolic syndrome are all part of the metabolic syndrome, which is intimately associated with insulin resistance. Additionally, it is a prelude to type 2 diabetes.

Symptoms and Signs:
Insulin resistance may not always present noticeable symptoms early on. Over time, increased hunger, fatigue, and difficulty losing weight may be observed. However, many individuals may be asymptomatic.

Diagnostic Tests:
Medical professionals use various tests to diagnose insulin resistance. Fasting blood sugar levels, fasting insulin levels, and the HbA1c test are common assessments that provide insights into insulin sensitivity.

Lifestyle Modifications:
Lifestyle changes play a pivotal role in managing insulin resistance. These changes include adopting a balanced diet, engaging in regular physical activity, managing stress, and maintaining a healthy weight.

Impact of Diet:
Dietary choices significantly influence insulin sensitivity. A diet rich in whole foods, low in processed sugars and refined carbohydrates, supports improved blood sugar regulation.

Physical Activity:
Regular physical activity enhances insulin sensitivity by promoting glucose uptake into muscles. Both aerobic exercises and strength training contribute to improved metabolic health.

Weight management: The key to controlling insulin resistance is to keep a healthy weight. Even a small amount of weight loss can make a big difference in improving insulin sensitivity.

Medical Interventions:
In some cases, medications may be prescribed to manage insulin resistance. These may include insulin-sensitizing drugs or medications to control blood sugar levels.

Preventive Strategies:
Adopting a proactive approach to prevent insulin resistance involves embracing a healthy lifestyle early on. This includes balanced nutrition, regular exercise, and maintaining a healthy weight.

Causes and Risk Factors

Insulin resistance results from a combination of genetic and lifestyle factors, creating a complex interplay that influences metabolic health. Here's an exploration of the causes and risk factors contributing to insulin resistance:

Genetic Predisposition:
Genetics play a significant role in insulin resistance. Individuals with a family history of type 2 diabetes or metabolic conditions may have a higher genetic predisposition.

Obesity:
Excess body weight, especially visceral fat around the abdomen, is a major risk factor for insulin resistance. Adipose tissue releases substances that can interfere with insulin's action.

Sedentary Lifestyle:
Lack of physical activity is a key contributor.
Regular exercise helps muscles use glucose
efficiently, promoting insulin sensitivity.
Sedentary behavior increases the risk of insulin
resistance.

Unhealthy Dietary Choices:
Diets high in refined sugars, processed
carbohydrates, and saturated fats contribute to
insulin resistance. These foods can lead to
obesity and interfere with the body's ability to
regulate blood sugar.

Age:
Aging is associated with a natural decline in
insulin sensitivity. As individuals age,
maintaining a healthy lifestyle becomes
increasingly crucial to counteract this decline.

Hormonal Changes:
Conditions associated with hormonal changes, such as polycystic ovary syndrome (PCOS) in women, can increase the risk of insulin resistance. Hormonal imbalances can disrupt normal insulin function.

Sleep Deprivation:
Inadequate or poor-quality sleep is linked to insulin resistance. Sleep deprivation can disrupt hormonal balance, affecting insulin sensitivity and increasing the risk of metabolic disturbances.

Stress:
Chronic stress activates the body's "fight or flight" response, leading to increased cortisol levels. Elevated cortisol can contribute to insulin resistance over time.

Inflammation:

Chronic inflammation is associated with insulin resistance. Conditions like obesity, poor diet, and sedentary behavior can promote inflammation, interfering with insulin signaling.

Smoking and Excessive Alcohol Consumption:

Smoking and excessive alcohol intake are linked to insulin resistance. These behaviors can negatively impact overall health, contributing to metabolic disturbances.

Medications:

Certain medications, such as glucocorticoids used to treat inflammatory conditions, can induce insulin resistance as a side effect. It's important to discuss potential impacts on insulin sensitivity with healthcare providers.

Environmental Factors:
Environmental factors, including exposure to endocrine-disrupting chemicals, may contribute to insulin resistance. These substances can interfere with hormonal balance.

Understanding the causes and risk factors for insulin resistance is crucial for adopting preventive measures and making informed lifestyle choices. By addressing modifiable risk factors through a combination of healthy eating, regular physical activity, and stress management, individuals can mitigate the impact of insulin resistance and support overall metabolic well-being.

Identifying Signs and Symptoms

Insulin resistance often develops gradually, and its early stages may not exhibit overt symptoms. However, certain signs and symptoms may signal the presence of insulin resistance. Here's a guide to identifying potential indicators:

Increased Hunger:
Insulin resistance can lead to difficulty in utilizing glucose for energy, resulting in increased hunger even after meals.

Persistent Fatigue:
Despite adequate rest, individuals with insulin resistance may experience persistent fatigue. This can be linked to the inefficiency of glucose uptake by cells.

Difficulty Losing Weight:
Insulin resistance may hinder weight loss efforts, making it challenging to shed excess pounds, especially around the abdominal area.

Acanthosis Nigricans:
A darkening and thickening of the skin, particularly in skin folds or creases, known as acanthosis nigricans, can be a visible sign of insulin resistance.

Frequent Urination:
Insulin resistance can contribute to elevated blood sugar levels, leading to increased thirst and consequently, frequent urination.

Blurry Vision:
Fluctuations in blood sugar levels associated with insulin resistance may cause temporary changes in vision, such as blurriness.

Skin Tags:
The presence of small, soft growths on the
skin, known as skin tags, especially in the neck
or armpit areas, may be associated with insulin
resistance.

Polycystic Ovary Syndrome (PCOS):
Women with insulin resistance may experience
irregular menstrual cycles, infertility, and other
symptoms associated with PCOS.

Elevated Blood Pressure:
Insulin resistance is often linked to increased
blood pressure, contributing to the risk of
developing hypertension.

High Triglyceride Levels:
Insulin resistance can result in elevated levels
of triglycerides, a type of fat in the blood,
increasing the risk of cardiovascular issues.

Low HDL Cholesterol:
Individuals with insulin resistance may have lower levels of high-density lipoprotein (HDL) cholesterol, commonly known as "good" cholesterol.

Increased Waist Circumference:
A larger waist circumference, especially when compared to hip measurements, is associated with insulin resistance. It is often indicative of visceral fat accumulation.

Skin Discoloration:
Dark patches on the skin, particularly in body creases and folds, can be a manifestation of insulin resistance-related skin changes.

Elevated Fasting Blood Sugar Levels:
Regular monitoring of fasting blood sugar levels can reveal elevated levels, indicating impaired glucose regulation.

It's important to note that these signs and symptoms may not be exclusive to insulin resistance and can also be associated with other health conditions. Additionally, some individuals with insulin resistance may remain asymptomatic, emphasizing the importance of routine health check-ups and screenings. If you suspect insulin resistance or experience these signs, consulting with a healthcare professional for a comprehensive evaluation is recommended. Early identification and intervention are key to managing insulin resistance and preventing associated complications.

The Link Between Insulin and Blood Sugar

The relationship between insulin and blood sugar is a finely tuned orchestration crucial for maintaining optimal metabolic balance. Here's an exploration of this intricate connection:

Insulin Production:
The pancreas, an organ located behind the stomach, produces insulin. Specialized cells in the pancreas, known as beta cells, release insulin in response to elevated blood sugar levels.

Blood Sugar Regulation: During digestion, carbohydrates are converted to glucose, or sugar, when ingested. Blood sugar levels rise as glucose enters the bloodstream.

Insulin as a Key Player:
Insulin acts as a key that unlocks cells, allowing them to take in glucose from the bloodstream. This process is essential for cells to use glucose as a source of energy.

Glucose Uptake by Cells:
Insulin facilitates the uptake of glucose by cells, particularly muscle and fat cells. Once inside the cells, glucose undergoes various metabolic processes to produce energy.

Storage of Extra Glucose: Insulin not only aids in the absorption of glucose but also aids in the storage of extra glucose as glycogen in the muscles and liver. When more energy is required, this stored glycogen can be transformed back into glucose.

Maintaining Blood Sugar Levels:
Insulin plays a pivotal role in maintaining blood sugar levels within a narrow and healthy range. After a meal, insulin helps lower elevated blood sugar by facilitating glucose uptake and storage.

Insulin Resistance:
In individuals with insulin resistance, cells become less responsive to insulin's signals. This resistance hampers the efficient uptake of glucose, leading to persistently elevated blood sugar levels.

Compensatory Insulin Production:
To counteract insulin resistance, the pancreas often produces more insulin to maintain blood sugar control. However, over time, this compensatory mechanism may become insufficient.

Hyperglycemia:
When insulin is unable to effectively lower blood sugar levels, it can result in hyperglycemia – elevated levels of glucose in the bloodstream. Prolonged hyperglycemia is a hallmark of diabetes.

Implications for Type 2 Diabetes:
In type 2 diabetes, insulin resistance progresses, and the pancreas may struggle to produce enough insulin. This can lead to a chronic elevation of blood sugar levels, contributing to the development of diabetes.

Role in Metabolic Syndrome:
Insulin resistance is a central component of metabolic syndrome, a cluster of conditions including high blood pressure, abnormal cholesterol levels, and abdominal obesity.

Importance of Balance:
The delicate balance between insulin and blood sugar is crucial for overall health. Disruptions in this balance, such as insulin resistance, can contribute to metabolic disorders and increase the risk of cardiovascular complications.

Understanding the link between insulin and blood sugar provides insights into the intricate mechanisms that govern metabolic health. Maintaining this delicate balance through a healthy lifestyle, including balanced nutrition, regular physical activity, and weight management, is key to preventing insulin resistance and promoting overall well-being.

CHAPTER THREE

Principles of the Insulin Resistance Diet

The core principles of the Insulin Resistance Diet are making deliberate food decisions to control blood sugar levels and improve insulin sensitivity. The following are the main ideas that direct this strategy:

Balanced Macronutrients:
Emphasize a balanced intake of macronutrients – carbohydrates, proteins, and fats. This balance helps regulate blood sugar levels and provides sustained energy.

Complex Carbohydrates Over Refined Sugars:
Prioritize complex carbohydrates found in whole grains, legumes, and vegetables over refined sugars.

These foods release glucose more gradually, preventing rapid spikes in blood sugar. Consume foods high in dietary fiber, such as fruits, vegetables, and whole grains. Fiber improves insulin sensitivity and stabilizes blood sugar levels by slowing down the absorption of glucose.

Lean Proteins:
Include lean protein sources such as poultry, fish, beans, and legumes. Protein supports muscle health, provides a feeling of fullness, and has minimal impact on blood sugar.

Healthy Fats: Choose foods high in avocados, nuts, seeds, and olive oil, among other sources of healthy fats. These lipids improve general well-being without impairing insulin sensitivity.

Portion Control:
Practice portion control to manage caloric intake. Controlling portions aids in weight management, an important aspect of improving insulin sensitivity.

Develop conscious eating practices with mindful eating. During meals, pay attention to indications of hunger and fullness, enjoy every bite, and keep yourself from becoming distracted. Eating with awareness fosters a positive connection with food.

Regular Meal Timing:
Establish regular meal timing to provide a steady supply of nutrients throughout the day. Consistent meal patterns contribute to stable blood sugar levels.

Limit Processed Foods:
Minimize the consumption of processed foods,
which often contain added sugars, unhealthy
fats, and refined carbohydrates. Opt for whole,
minimally processed foods for a nutrient-dense
diet.

Low-Glycemic Foods:
Choose low-glycemic foods to help manage
blood sugar levels. These include non-starchy
vegetables, berries, and whole grains that have
a gradual impact on glucose.

Hydration: Drink water as your main beverage
to stay properly hydrated. Staying well
hydrated can help regulate hunger and
promote general health.

Moderate Alcohol Intake:
If consuming alcohol, do so in moderation.
Excessive alcohol intake can affect blood sugar
levels and overall metabolic health.

Regular Physical Activity:
Incorporate regular physical activity into your
routine. Both aerobic exercises and strength
training contribute to improved insulin
sensitivity.

Weight Management:
Maintain a healthy weight through a
combination of balanced nutrition and physical
activity. Weight management is crucial for
managing insulin resistance.

Individualized Approach:
Recognize the importance of individualization.
Dietary needs can vary, and factors such as
age, activity level, and underlying health
conditions should inform personalized dietary
choices.

Balancing Macronutrients

Balancing macronutrients is a fundamental aspect of managing insulin resistance, focusing on optimizing the intake of carbohydrates, proteins, and fats to support blood sugar regulation. Here's a closer look at how to achieve this balance:

Carbs: Prefer quality to quantity Give complex carbs—like those found in whole grains, legumes, and vegetables—priority over processed carbohydrates. Due to their lower glycemic index, these meals release glucose into the bloodstream more gradually and steadily, reducing the risk of sudden increases in blood sugar.

Fiber-Dense Optional: Select carbs with high fiber content to increase fullness and decrease glucose absorption. Whole grains, fruits, and vegetables are examples of foods high in fiber.

Proteins:

Lean Protein Sources: Include lean protein sources like poultry, fish, tofu, beans, and legumes. Protein supports muscle health, provides a feeling of fullness, and has a minimal impact on blood sugar levels.

Balanced Distribution: Distribute protein intake evenly throughout the day, including it in each meal. This helps maintain a steady supply of amino acids and supports overall metabolic function.

Fats:

Healthy Fat Choices: Opt for healthy fats, such as avocados, nuts, seeds, and olive oil. These fats contribute to overall health and do not negatively affect insulin sensitivity.

Portion Control: While healthy fats are beneficial, portion control is essential. Monitor serving sizes to manage caloric intake.

Meal Timing:
Consistent Timing: Establish regular meal timing to create a predictable pattern for nutrient intake. Consistency in meal timing supports stable blood sugar levels and aids in insulin sensitivity.
Balanced Meals and Snacks: Plan balanced meals and snacks throughout the day. Combining carbohydrates with proteins and fats in each meal helps modulate the impact on blood sugar.

Water as the Main Drink for Hydration: Drink plenty of water as your main hydration source. Maintaining adequate hydration promotes general health and may help regulate hunger.
Limit beverages high in sugar: Reduce the amount of sugar-filled beverages you consume because they can cause sharp rises in blood sugar. Drink water, herbal teas, or other calorie-efficient beverages.

Individualization:
Tailored Approach: Recognize that individual nutritional needs may vary. Consider factors such as age, activity level, and underlying health conditions when customizing macronutrient intake.
Monitoring and Adjusting: Regularly monitor blood sugar levels and assess how different macronutrient ratios impact individual responses. Adjust the balance as needed based on these observations.

Balancing macronutrients for insulin resistance involves a thoughtful and personalized approach. It's advisable to work with healthcare professionals or registered dietitians to create an individualized meal plan that aligns with specific health goals and considerations. By incorporating a balanced mix of carbohydrates, proteins, and fats, individuals can promote stable blood sugar levels and support overall metabolic health.

Understanding Glycemic Index

The Glycemic Index (GI) is a valuable tool in managing insulin resistance, providing insights into how different carbohydrates affect blood sugar levels. Here's a breakdown of understanding the Glycemic Index and its relevance:

Definition of the Glycemic Index: The Glycemic Index is a rating system that uses numbers to indicate how different types of carbohydrates affect blood sugar levels. Foods with a higher GI raise blood sugar levels more quickly and significantly, whole foods with a lower GI raise blood sugar levels more gradually and more slowly.

GI Scale:

Low GI (0-55): Foods with a low GI are digested and absorbed more slowly, resulting in a gradual increase in blood sugar. Examples include most non-starchy vegetables, legumes, and certain whole grains.

Medium GI (56-69): Foods in this range have a moderate impact on blood sugar. Examples include whole wheat products and some fruits.

High GI (70 and above): Foods with a high GI cause a rapid spike in blood sugar levels. Examples include refined sugars, white bread, and certain cereals.

Relevance to Insulin Resistance:

Preventing Spikes: For individuals with insulin resistance, avoiding rapid spikes in blood sugar is crucial. Choosing foods with a lower GI can help achieve more stable blood sugar levels and enhance insulin sensitivity.

Managing Insulin Response: Low-GI foods promote a slower release of glucose into the bloodstream, reducing the need for a rapid and excessive insulin response. This is particularly beneficial for those with insulin resistance.

Selecting Low-GI Foods:
Non-Starchy Vegetables: Most non-starchy vegetables, such as broccoli, spinach, and peppers, have a low GI.
Legumes: Beans, lentils, and chickpeas are excellent sources of low-GI carbohydrates.
Whole Grains: Choose whole grains like quinoa, barley, and oats over refined grains for lower-GI options.
Fruits: Opt for fruits with a lower GI, such as berries, cherries, and apples.

Combining Foods for Balanced GI:
Balanced Meals: Creating balanced meals that include a combination of low-GI carbohydrates, lean proteins, and healthy fats can help moderate the overall GI of the meal.

Fiber Content: Foods high in fiber tend to have a lower GI. Fiber slows down digestion and the absorption of glucose.

Considerations:
Individual Variability: The GI of foods can vary between individuals, and factors such as cooking methods, ripeness, and food combinations can influence the overall impact on blood sugar.
Glycemic Load (GL): While GI is a useful tool, considering the Glycemic Load provides a more comprehensive picture by accounting for both the quality and quantity of carbohydrates consumed.

Understanding and incorporating the Glycemic Index into meal planning can be a valuable strategy for managing insulin resistance. By choosing low-GI foods and adopting a balanced approach to meals, individuals can promote stable blood sugar levels and support overall metabolic health.

Portion Control and Meal Timing

Effectively managing insulin resistance involves not only choosing the right foods but also paying attention to when and how much you eat. Here's a guide to the principles of portion control and meal timing for an insulin resistance diet:

Portion Control:

Balanced Serving Sizes: Be mindful of portion sizes to avoid overeating. Balance your plate with appropriate servings of carbohydrates, proteins, and fats to prevent excessive caloric intake.

Use Visual Cues: Use visual cues to estimate portions. For example, a serving of lean protein is about the size of your palm, and a serving of carbohydrates (like rice or pasta) should be around the size of your fist.

Plate Method: Adopt the plate method by dividing your plate into sections for vegetables, lean protein, and whole grains. This naturally promotes a balanced and portion-controlled meal.

Time of Meals: Typical Meal Plan: Set up a regular mealtime schedule that is consistent. This promotes the body's normal insulin response and aids in blood sugar regulation.
Avoid Skipping Meals: Skipping meals can cause blood sugar levels to fluctuate and may encourage overeating at other times. Try to eat three well-balanced meals a day, and add in some nutritious snacks in between if necessary.
Consciously Consuming Food: Observe your body's signals of hunger and fullness. Consume food only when you're hungry and quit when you're full. By being mindful, overeating can be avoided.

Prevent Eating Late at Night: Eat less late at night because the body's sensitivity to insulin tends to decline in the evening. In order to allow for adequate digestion, finish meals at least a few hours before going to bed.

Balancing Nutrients in Each Meal:
Carbohydrates with Proteins and Fats: Include a combination of carbohydrates, proteins, and healthy fats in each meal. This balanced approach slows down the absorption of glucose, promoting stable blood sugar levels. **Fiber-Rich Foods:** Prioritize fiber-rich foods, such as vegetables, fruits, and whole grains. Fiber contributes to satiety and helps control blood sugar levels.

Stopping Blood Sugar Increases:
Refined carbs should be limited. Reduce your intake of processed sugars and carbs because they can quickly raise your blood sugar levels. Select complete, unprocessed foods to achieve long-lasting energy.
Glycemic Index Knowledge: Think about the food glycemic index. Choose low-GI foods to avoid unexpected spikes in blood sugar.

Hydration Timing:
Hydrate Before Meals: Drink water before meals to help control appetite and prevent overeating. Sometimes, feelings of thirst can be mistaken for hunger.
Limit Sugary Drinks: Minimize the intake of sugary beverages, as they can contribute to blood sugar fluctuations.

Post-Meal Activity:

Light Physical Activity: Consider engaging in light physical activity, like a short walk, after meals. This can aid in glucose metabolism and improve insulin sensitivity.

By incorporating portion control and strategic meal timing into your routine, you can optimize the nutritional impact on blood sugar levels. These practices contribute to a balanced insulin resistance diet, promoting metabolic health and overall well-being. As always, personalized advice from healthcare professionals or registered dietitians can enhance the effectiveness of these strategies based on individual needs and health status.

CHAPTER FOUR

Setting Up Your Kitchen for Success

Creating a kitchen environment that aligns with your insulin resistance dietary goals involves thoughtful organization, strategic choices, and easy access to nutritious ingredients. Here's a guide on setting up your kitchen for success:

Keeping Whole, High-Nutrient Foods on Hand:

Fresh Vegetables: Have a wide selection of fresh fruits and veggies on hand. It takes these foods high in fiber to support stable blood sugar levels.

entire Grains: Keep entire grains on hand, such as oats, brown rice, and quinoa. If you want a slower release of glucose, choose them over refined grains.

Lean Proteins: Always keep lean protein sources on available, including fish, poultry, tofu, and lentils. Proteins enhance muscular health and aid promote satiety.

Consume foods high in unsaturated fats, such as olive oil, avocados, almonds, and seeds. These fats can be included in a balanced diet to address insulin resistance and promote general health.

Organizing Your Pantry:

Low-Glycemic Snacks: Keep low-glycemic snacks handy, such as nuts, seeds, and whole grain crackers. These can be convenient choices for satisfying hunger between meals.

Canned Legumes: Stock up on canned legumes like chickpeas and black beans for quick and easy protein additions to salads or meals.

Smart Carbohydrate Choices:
Whole Grain Options: Choose whole grain alternatives for staples like bread, pasta, and rice. Look for labels indicating whole grains as the primary ingredient.
Alternative Flours: Experiment with alternative flours like almond flour or coconut flour for baking to reduce the glycemic impact of your recipes.

Meal Prep Tools:
Portion-Controlled Containers: Invest in portion-controlled containers for meal prepping. This makes it easier to control serving sizes and have balanced meals readily available.
Batch Cooking: Consider batch cooking and freezing portions. Having pre-prepared, balanced meals can save time and prevent resorting to less healthy options on busy days.

Smart Snacking Options:
Cut-Up Vegetables: Prepare cut-up vegetables in advance for quick and healthy snacking. Pair them with hummus or a yogurt-based dip for added protein.
Fresh Fruit Bowls: Keep a bowl of fresh fruit on the counter for a convenient and visually appealing snack option.

Hydration Station:
Water Accessibility: Make water easily accessible. Keep a water bottle with you throughout the day to stay hydrated and help control appetite.
Herbal Teas: Explore herbal teas as a low-calorie beverage option. Some teas, like cinnamon tea, may have additional benefits for blood sugar regulation.

Limiting Processed Foods:
Minimize Processed Snacks: Reduce the availability of processed snacks high in sugars and refined carbohydrates. Instead, focus on whole, nutrient-dense options.

Educational Resources:
Cookbooks and Resources: Have insulin resistance-friendly cookbooks and educational resources in your kitchen. These can provide inspiration and guidance for preparing balanced meals.

Kitchen Tools for Healthy Cooking:
Non-Stick Pans: Invest in non-stick pans to reduce the need for excessive cooking oils.
Steamer Baskets: Use a steamer basket for cooking vegetables while preserving their nutritional content.

Label Awareness:
Read Nutrition Labels: Develop the habit of reading nutrition labels to identify hidden sugars and make informed choices.

Supportive Kitchen Gadgets:
Food Scale: Use a food scale for accurate portion measurements.
Blender or Food Processor: Incorporate these for smoothies or homemade sauces, allowing control over ingredients.

By creating a kitchen environment that supports your insulin resistance dietary goals, you set yourself up for success in making healthier choices. A well-organized and stocked kitchen encourages mindful eating and makes it easier to adhere to your nutritional plan. Always consult with healthcare professionals or registered dietitians for personalized advice based on your specific needs and health status.

Stocking a Diabetes-Friendly Pantry

The process of creating an insulin resistance-friendly pantry for diabetics includes choosing healthful, high-nutrient items that support stable blood sugar levels. This is a thorough guide on filling your pantry:

Whole Grains:
Quinoa: A versatile and protein-rich whole grain.
Brown Rice: A fiber-packed alternative to white rice.
Oats: A great source of soluble fiber to support heart health.

Legumes:
Black Beans, Chickpeas, Lentils: High in fiber and protein, they have a low glycemic index.

Healthy Fats:
Olive Oil: A heart-healthy oil for cooking and dressing.
Nuts and Seeds: Almonds, walnuts, chia seeds, and flax seeds provide healthy fats and fiber.

Lean Proteins:
Chicken Breast, Turkey, Fish: Lean protein sources for muscle health.
Tofu and Tempeh: Plant-based protein options.

Low-Glycemic Sweeteners:
Stevia, Erythritol, Monk Fruit: Natural sweeteners with minimal impact on blood sugar.

Herbs and Spices:
Cinnamon, Turmeric, Garlic, Ginger: Flavorful additions with potential blood sugar benefits.

Whole Vegetables and Fruits:
Leafy Greens, Broccoli, Bell Peppers:
Nutrient-dense vegetables.
Berries, Apples, Pears: Low-glycemic fruits rich in antioxidants.

Whole Grain Products:
Whole Wheat Pasta, Whole Grain Bread:
Fibrous alternatives to refined grains.

Low-Sodium Canned Goods:
Tomatoes, Beans, Tuna: Versatile ingredients with reduced sodium content.

Dairy or Dairy Alternatives:
Greek Yogurt, Almond Milk: Protein-rich and low in added sugars.

Eggs:
A protein source versatile for various dishes.

Nutrient-Dense Snacks:
Raw Vegetables with Hummus: A satisfying
and low-carb snack.
Nuts and Seeds Mix: A portable and
energy-boosting option.

Whole Grain Cereals:
Oatmeal, Bran Flakes: High-fiber choices with
minimal added sugars.

Broths and Stocks:
Low-Sodium Chicken or Vegetable Broth: For
flavorful and low-calorie soups.

Flour Alternatives:
Almond Flour, Coconut Flour: Lower-carb
options for baking.

Canned Fish:
Salmon, Sardines: Rich in omega-3 fatty
acids for heart health.

Vinegar:
Apple Cider Vinegar: Adds flavor without added sugars and may have potential health benefits.

Tea and Coffee:
Green Tea, Herbal Tea, Black Coffee: Low-calorie beverage options.

Unsweetened Applesauce:
A natural sweetener substitute in recipes.

Dark Chocolate (70% Cocoa or Higher):
A moderate indulgence with potential antioxidant benefits.

Essential Ingredients for Insulin-Friendly Cooking

Creating insulin-friendly meals involves selecting ingredients that support stable blood sugar levels and overall metabolic health. Here's a list of essential ingredients for insulin-friendly cooking:

Whole Grains:
Quinoa, Brown Rice, Oats: High-fiber whole grains with a lower glycemic index.

Lean Proteins:
Chicken Breast, Turkey, Fish: Lean sources of protein for muscle health.
Tofu, Tempeh: Plant-based protein alternatives.

Heart-healthy fats for flavor and satiety are avocado and olive oil.
Nuts and Seeds: Walnuts, almonds, chia seeds, and flaxseeds are good sources of extra nutrients and good fats.

Low-Glycemic Vegetables:
Leafy Greens, Broccoli, Cauliflower:
Non-starchy vegetables rich in fiber and
vitamins.
Bell Peppers, Zucchini, Tomatoes: Colorful
additions with a lower impact on blood sugar.

Berries:
Blueberries, Strawberries, Raspberries:
Low-glycemic fruits rich in antioxidants.

Herbs and Spices:
Cinnamon, Turmeric, Garlic, Ginger:
Flavorful additions with potential blood sugar
benefits.

Low-Glycemic Fruits:
Apples, Pears, Cherries: Fruits that provide
natural sweetness without rapid blood sugar
spikes.

Whole Grain Products:
Whole Wheat Pasta, Quinoa Pasta, Brown
Rice Noodles: Fiber-rich alternatives to refined
grains.

Greek Yogurt or Dairy Alternatives:
Low-Fat Greek Yogurt, Almond Milk:
Protein-rich and lower in added sugars.

Legumes:
Black Beans, Chickpeas, Lentils: High-fiber
sources of plant-based protein.

Eggs:
A versatile and protein-packed ingredient.

Salmon or Fatty Fish:
Rich in omega-3 fatty acids for heart health.
Non-Starchy Vegetables for
Snacking:
Carrot Sticks, Cucumber Slices, Cherry
Tomatoes: Convenient and healthy snack
options.

Flavorful Vinegars:
Balsamic Vinegar, Apple Cider Vinegar: Add flavor without added sugars.

Low-Sodium Broths:
Chicken or Vegetable Broth: Base for flavorful and low-calorie soups.

Alternative Flours:
Almond Flour, Coconut Flour: Lower-carb options for baking.

Dark Chocolate (70% Cocoa or Higher):
A moderate indulgence with potential antioxidant benefits.

Herbal Teas and Unsweetened Coffee:
Green Tea, Chamomile Tea, Black Coffee: Low-calorie beverage options.

Spaghetti Squash or Zucchini Noodles:
Low-carb alternatives to traditional pasta.

Garbanzo Bean Flour (Chickpea Flour):
A gluten-free, high-protein alternative for
baking.

By incorporating these essential ingredients
into your cooking, you can craft well-balanced
and nutrient-dense meals that support
insulin-friendly nutrition. Experiment with
different combinations, cooking methods, and
recipes to find what suits your taste
preferences and dietary needs. Additionally,
seeking guidance from healthcare
professionals or registered dietitians can help
tailor your meal plans to your specific health
goals and requirements.

Smart Shopping Tips

Make a shopping list based on your intended dishes and plan your meals and snacks for the coming week. This aids in maintaining attention and preventing impulsive purchases.

Shop the Perimeter:
Fresh Produce, Lean Proteins, Dairy: The perimeter of the store often contains whole, fresh foods. Focus on items like fruits, vegetables, lean meats, and dairy.

Select Whole Foods:
Reduce Prepared Foods: Choose unprocessed or minimally processed foods. These products usually have less processed carbs and added sugars.

Read Nutrition Labels:
Check Carbohydrate Content: Examine
nutrition labels for total carbohydrate content,
especially sugars and fiber. Choose products
with higher fiber and lower sugar.

Glycemic Index Awareness:
Select Low-Glycemic Options: Prioritize
foods with a low glycemic index. These options
have a slower impact on blood sugar levels.

Fresh Produce Selection:
Colorful Variety: Choose a variety of colorful
fruits and vegetables. The diverse range
ensures a mix of nutrients and antioxidants.

Lean Proteins: Fish, Poultry, and Plant-Based
Foods Choose sources of lean protein.
Legumes, fish, poultry, and tofu are all great
options.

Healthy Fats:
Avocado, Nuts, Olive Oil: Incorporate sources
of healthy fats. Avocados, nuts, and olive oil
are nutritious additions.

Dairy or Alternatives:
Low-Fat Greek Yogurt, Unsweetened Almond
Milk: Opt for low-fat or non-fat dairy options.
Consider unsweetened almond milk as an
alternative.

Whole Grain Products:
Whole Wheat, Quinoa, Brown Rice: Choose
whole grain alternatives for bread, pasta, and
rice.

Herbs and Spices:
Cinnamon, Turmeric, Garlic: Enhance flavor
with herbs and spices. Some, like cinnamon,
may have additional health benefits.

Avoid Sugary Drinks:
Choose Water, Herbal Tea: Minimize sugary
beverage purchases. Water and herbal teas
are healthier options.

Limit Processed Snacks:
Opt for Nutrient-Dense Snacks: Reduce the
temptation to buy processed snacks high in
sugars. Instead, choose nuts, seeds, or fresh
fruits.

Check for Hidden Sugars:
Read Ingredient Lists: Be vigilant for hidden
sugars in ingredient lists. Different names for
sugar include sucrose, high fructose corn
syrup, and agave nectar.

Compare Brands:
Review Nutrition Labels: Compare nutrition
labels between brands to make informed
choices. Select products with better nutritional
profiles.

Shopping with a Full Stomach:
Avoid Impulse Buys: Shop after a meal to resist the urge to buy unnecessary, less healthy items when hungry.

Utilize Online Resources:
Nutrition Apps and Websites: Use online resources to check nutrition information and glycemic index values before shopping.

Buy in Bulk for Staples:
Grains, Legumes, Nuts: Purchase staples like whole grains, legumes, and nuts in bulk to save money and ensure a steady supply.

Be Mindful of Portions:
Select Individual Portions: When buying snacks or pre-packaged items, opt for individually portioned servings to manage intake.

Stay Informed:
Stay Updated on Nutrition Information: Keep abreast of nutritional guidelines and updates to make informed choices.

By incorporating these smart shopping tips, you can navigate the grocery store with a focus on insulin-friendly foods, supporting your efforts to maintain stable blood sugar levels and promote overall metabolic health.

CHAPTER FIVE

Equipping Your Kitchen with the Right Tools

Food Scale:
Purpose: Accurately measure portion sizes for precise carbohydrate, protein, and fat control.

Measuring Cups and Spoons:
Purpose: Ensure accurate measurements of ingredients, especially for baking or cooking specific recipes.

Steamer Basket:
Purpose: Retain the nutritional content of vegetables by steaming, a cooking method that helps maintain insulin-friendly qualities.

Non-Stick Pans:
Purpose: Minimize the need for excessive cooking oils while preparing meals, supporting a lower-fat cooking approach.

Blender or Food Processor:
Purpose: Create smoothies or homemade sauces with control over ingredients, facilitating nutrient-dense and insulin-friendly options.

Portion-Controlled Containers:
Purpose: Assist in meal prepping by providing controlled portions, promoting balanced and mindful eating.

Vegetable Spiralizer:
Purpose: Transform vegetables into low-carb alternatives for traditional pasta, promoting a lower-glycemic approach.

Quality Knives:
Purpose: Ensure efficient and safe food preparation, facilitating the inclusion of a variety of fresh produce.

Herb and Spice Grinder:
Purpose: Utilize fresh herbs and spices for flavor enhancement without relying on excessive salt or sugar.

Baking Sheets and Muffin Tins:
Purpose: Support healthier baking options with the ability to control ingredients in insulin-friendly recipes.

Slow Cooker or Instant Pot:
Purpose: Create nutritious and balanced meals with minimal effort, allowing for long, slow cooking that enhances flavors.

Salad Spinner:
Purpose: Easily prepare salads with fresh greens, promoting a diet rich in fiber and essential nutrients.

Citrus Juicer:
Purpose: Extract fresh juice from citrus fruits without added sugars, enhancing the flavor of dishes and beverages.

Water Filtration System:
Purpose: Ensure access to clean and refreshing water, promoting hydration without the need for sugary drinks.

Cutting Boards:
Purpose: Separate boards for different food groups, preventing cross-contamination and promoting food safety.

Nut Milk Bag:
Purpose: Make homemade nut milks or strain liquids, offering a lower-calorie alternative to traditional dairy.

Digital Thermometer:
Purpose: Ensure meats are cooked to the proper temperature for safety and flavor, supporting lean protein choices.

Vegetable Peeler:
Purpose: Quickly prepare vegetables for cooking or snacking, promoting the inclusion of nutrient-dense options.

Digital Timer:
Purpose: Assist in precise cooking times, preventing overcooking or undercooking and ensuring optimal taste and texture.

Sous Vide Precision Cooker:
Purpose: Cook meats precisely at lower temperatures, preserving tenderness and nutritional quality.

Having these tools in your kitchen can enhance your ability to prepare and enjoy insulin-friendly meals. They promote efficient cooking methods, portion control, and creativity in adapting recipes to suit your dietary needs. Always remember to consult with healthcare professionals or registered dietitians for personalized advice and guidance based on your specific health goals and requirements.

Cooking Oils and Ingredients to Embrace or Avoid

Extra Virgin Olive Oil (EVOO):
Embrace: Rich in monounsaturated fats and antioxidants, EVOO supports heart health and may improve insulin sensitivity.

Avocado Oil:
Embrace: High in monounsaturated fats, avocado oil provides a source of healthy fats without contributing to insulin resistance.

Coconut Oil (in Moderation):
Embrace: While high in saturated fats, coconut oil can be used in moderation for its potential anti-inflammatory properties.

Walnut Oil:
Embrace: Contains omega-3 fatty acids and antioxidants, contributing to heart health and potential insulin sensitivity.

Flaxseed Oil:
Embrace: Rich in omega-3 fatty acids,
flaxseed oil supports overall health and may
have anti-inflammatory effects.

Sesame Oil:
Embrace: Provides a distinct flavor and
contains healthy fats, adding variety to
insulin-friendly dishes.

Ghee or Clarified Butter:
Embrace (in moderation): While a source of
saturated fats, ghee is low in lactose and may
be tolerated by those sensitive to dairy.

Grass-Fed Butter:
Embrace (in moderation): Contains omega-3
fatty acids and CLA, contributing to potential
health benefits.

Herbs and Spices:
Embrace: Use herbs and spices liberally for flavor without added salt or sugar. Examples include cinnamon, turmeric, garlic, and ginger.

Apple Cider Vinegar:
Embrace: May have potential blood sugar-lowering effects and can be used as a flavorful alternative to traditional vinegars.

Balsamic Vinegar (in moderation):
Embrace: Adds flavor without added sugars when used in moderation.

Dijon Mustard:
Embrace: Low in calories and sugar, Dijon mustard provides flavor without negatively impacting blood sugar.

Ingredients to Avoid for Insulin Resistance Diet Cookbook:

Refined Sugar:
Avoid: High intake of refined sugars contributes to blood sugar spikes.

High-Fructose Corn Syrup (HFCS):
Avoid: Common in processed foods, HFCS can lead to insulin resistance when consumed in excess.

White Flour:
Avoid: Lacks fiber and nutrients, causing rapid increases in blood sugar levels.

Processed Foods:
Avoid: Often contain hidden sugars, unhealthy fats, and artificial additives.

Trans Fats:
Avoid: Found in partially hydrogenated oils, trans fats can contribute to inflammation and insulin resistance.

Excessive Saturated Fats:
Avoid (in excess): While some saturated fats are acceptable, excessive intake may contribute to insulin resistance.

Artificial Sweeteners (in Moderation):
Limit: Some studies suggest artificial sweeteners may impact gut bacteria and metabolism; use in moderation.

Highly Processed Cooking Oils:
Avoid: Oils high in omega-6 fatty acids, like soybean and corn oil, may contribute to inflammation.

MSG (Monosodium Glutamate):
Avoid: Commonly found in processed foods, MSG may have negative effects on insulin sensitivity.

Hidden Sugars in Condiments:
Avoid: Check labels for added sugars in condiments like ketchup, barbecue sauce, and salad dressings.

Excessive Salt:
Limit: High sodium intake can contribute to hypertension, which may affect insulin sensitivity.

In creating an insulin resistance diet cookbook, emphasize whole, unprocessed foods, lean proteins, and healthy fats. Use cooking oils and ingredients that contribute to overall health while avoiding those that may negatively impact blood sugar levels and insulin sensitivity. Always consult with healthcare professionals or registered dietitians for personalized advice based on individual health needs and goals.

CHAPTER SIX

Crafting Balanced Meals

Protein-Rich Foundation:
Why: Proteins stabilize blood sugar levels and promote satiety.
Examples: Lean meats, poultry, fish, tofu, legumes.

Fiber-Filled Vegetables:
Why: Fiber slows the absorption of glucose, preventing rapid blood sugar spikes.
Examples: Leafy greens, broccoli, cauliflower, bell peppers.

Slow-Release Carbohydrates:
Why: Choose complex carbohydrates to avoid sudden glucose surges.
Examples: Quinoa, brown rice, sweet potatoes, whole grains.

Healthy Fats for Satiety:
Why: Fats contribute to a feeling of fullness
and support overall health.
Examples: Avocado, olive oil, nuts, seeds.

Portion Control:
Why: Managing portion sizes helps control
calorie intake and blood sugar levels.
Tip: Use smaller plates and be mindful of
serving sizes.

Balanced Snacking:
Why: Snacks with a mix of protein, fiber, and
healthy fats maintain steady energy levels.
Examples: Greek yogurt with berries, raw
veggies with hummus.

Mindful Carb Choices:
Why: Opt for low-glycemic carbs to minimize
blood sugar fluctuations.
Examples: Berries, whole fruits, non-starchy
vegetables.

Herbs and Spices for Flavor:
Why: Enhance taste without added salt, sugar, or calories.
Examples: Cinnamon, turmeric, garlic, ginger.

Hydration Importance:
Why: Water supports metabolism and aids in digestion.
Tip: Stay hydrated with water; limit sugary drinks.

Meal Timing and Consistency:
Why: Regular meals and snacks help maintain stable blood sugar levels.
Tip: Aim for consistency in meal timing.

Limit Processed Foods:
Why: Processed foods often contain hidden sugars and unhealthy fats.
Tip: Choose whole, unprocessed options whenever possible.

Include Omega-3 Fatty Acids:
Why: Omega-3s may have anti-inflammatory effects and support heart health.
Examples: Fatty fish (salmon, trout), chia seeds, flaxseeds.

Prefer Low-Glycemic Sweeteners:
Why: Choose sweeteners with a lower impact on blood sugar levels.
Examples: Stevia, erythritol, monk fruit.

Monitor Alcohol Intake:
Why: Alcohol can affect blood sugar; moderation is key.
Tip: If consuming, do so with food and limit quantities.

Regular Physical Activity:
Why: Exercise improves insulin sensitivity and aids in weight management.
Tip: Engage in activities you enjoy regularly.

Mindful Eating Practices:
Why: Being present during meals helps avoid overeating.
Tip: Eat slowly, savor each bite, and listen to hunger cues.

Consultation with Healthcare Professionals:
Why: Personalized advice from healthcare providers or dietitians ensures tailored strategies for individual needs.

Balanced meals for insulin resistance prioritize a combination of proteins, fibers, and healthy fats while managing portion sizes and choosing nutrient-dense ingredients. Consistency, mindful eating, and incorporating a variety of foods contribute to overall stability in blood sugar levels. Always seek personalized advice from healthcare professionals or registered dietitians based on individual health conditions and goals.

Building a Nutrient-Rich Plate

Fill Half Your Plate with Non-Starchy Vegetables:
Why: Rich in fiber, vitamins, and minerals; they have a minimal impact on blood sugar.
Examples: Leafy greens, broccoli, cauliflower, bell peppers.

Give Lean Proteins a Quarter of Your Plate:
Reason: Proteins help to sate hunger and maintain blood sugar levels.
Turkey, salmon, tofu, lentils, and chicken breast are a few examples.

Dedicate a Quarter of Your Plate to Whole Grains or Low-Glycemic Carbs:
Why: Complex carbs provide sustained energy without causing rapid blood sugar spikes.
Examples: Quinoa, brown rice, sweet potatoes, whole grains.

Incorporate Healthy Fats:
Why: Fats support overall health and enhance the feeling of fullness.
Examples: Avocado, olive oil, nuts, seeds.

Add Color and Flavor with Herbs and Spices:
Why: Enhance taste without added salt, sugar, or calories.
Examples: Cinnamon, turmeric, garlic, ginger.

Include Omega-3 Fatty Acids:
Why: Omega-3s have anti-inflammatory effects and contribute to heart health.
Examples: Fatty fish (salmon, trout), chia seeds, flaxseeds.

Choose Low-Glycemic Sweeteners:
Why: Opt for sweeteners with minimal impact on blood sugar levels.
Examples: Stevia, erythritol, monk fruit.

Stay Hydrated with Water:
Why: Water supports metabolism and aids in digestion without added calories.
Tip: Prioritize water as your main beverage.

Consider Portion Control:
Why: Managing portion sizes helps control calorie intake and blood sugar levels.
Tip: Use smaller plates and be mindful of serving sizes.

Limit Processed Foods:
Why: Processed foods often contain hidden sugars and unhealthy fats.
Tip: Choose whole, unprocessed options whenever possible.

Moderate Alcohol Intake:
Why: Alcohol can impact blood sugar; moderation is key.
Tip: If consuming, do so with food and limit quantities.

Monitor and Record Food Choices:
Why: Keeping a food diary helps track choices and identify patterns.
Tip: Use a journal or a nutrition app for accurate records.

Include Regular Physical Activity:
Why: Exercise improves insulin sensitivity and aids in weight management.
Tip: Engage in activities you enjoy regularly.

Practice Mindful Eating:
Why: Being present during meals helps avoid overeating.
Tip: Eat slowly, savor each bite, and listen to hunger cues.

Consultation with Healthcare Professionals:
Why: Personalized advice from healthcare providers or dietitians ensures tailored strategies for individual needs.

Building a nutrient-rich plate for insulin resistance involves a thoughtful combination of non-starchy vegetables, lean proteins, whole grains, healthy fats, and mindful eating practices. Consistency, variety, and personalized guidance contribute to overall well-being and effective blood sugar management. Always seek advice from healthcare professionals or registered dietitians based on individual health conditions and goals.

Creating Balanced Meals for Blood Sugar Control

Creating balanced meals for blood sugar control involves careful consideration of the types and amounts of nutrients to maintain stable glucose levels. Here's a comprehensive breakdown:

Carbohydrates:
Choose complex carbohydrates like whole grains (brown rice, quinoa, oats) over refined grains.
Monitor portion sizes to control the amount of carbohydrates consumed.
Prioritize high-fiber foods, as they slow down digestion and reduce blood sugar spikes.

Proteins:
Include lean protein sources such as poultry,
fish, tofu, beans, and legumes.
Protein helps stabilize blood sugar and
promotes a feeling of fullness, preventing
overeating.

Fats: Choose heart-healthy fats from foods like
olive oil, avocados, almonds, and seeds.
Reduce the amount of trans and saturated fats
in processed snacks and fried foods.

Fruits and Vegetables:
Emphasize a variety of colorful, non-starchy
vegetables and moderate portions of fruits.
These provide essential vitamins, minerals,
and antioxidants without causing rapid spikes
in blood sugar.

Meal Timing:
Distribute meals throughout the day with
balanced portions to prevent extreme
fluctuations in blood sugar.
Include snacks if necessary to maintain
consistent energy levels.

Portion Control:
Be mindful of portion sizes to avoid overeating
and better manage blood sugar levels.
Use smaller plates to help control portions
visually.

Hydration:
Drink plenty of water throughout the day to stay
hydrated, which supports overall health and
can aid in blood sugar regulation.

Avoid Sugary Beverages:
Limit or avoid sugary drinks like sodas and fruit
juices, as they can cause rapid spikes in blood
sugar.

Regular Monitoring:
Monitor blood sugar levels regularly to understand how different foods impact your body.
Adjust your diet based on your individual responses and consult healthcare professionals for guidance.

Customization:
Consider individual factors such as age, activity level, and any existing health conditions when tailoring meals for blood sugar control.
Consult with healthcare professionals or a registered dietitian for personalized advice and meal plans.

Remember, creating balanced meals is not a one-size-fits-all approach, and it's crucial to adapt dietary choices based on individual needs and responses.

Incorporating Colorful Vegetables and Fruits

Including a variety of vibrant fruits and vegetables in an insulin resistance diet is helpful for controlling blood sugar levels and supplying vital minerals, antioxidants, and fiber. Here is a thorough how-to:

Color Variety:
Aim for a diverse range of colors in your fruits and vegetables, as different hues often indicate various phytonutrients with unique health benefits.

Dark Leafy Greens:
Include kale, spinach, collard greens, and Swiss chard, which are rich in vitamins, minerals, and antioxidants. These low-calorie options have a minimal impact on blood sugar.

Brightly Colored Berries:
Berries like blueberries, strawberries, raspberries, and blackberries are rich in fiber, vitamins, and antioxidants. They have a lower glycemic index, minimizing blood sugar spikes.

Citrus Fruits:
Oranges, grapefruits, lemons, and limes provide vitamin C, fiber, and antioxidants. Opt for whole fruits rather than fruit juices to maintain fiber content.

Cruciferous Vegetables:
Broccoli, cauliflower, Brussels sprouts, and cabbage are excellent choices. They contain fiber, vitamins, and compounds that support detoxification processes in the body.

Colorful Bell Peppers:
Include red, yellow, and green bell peppers for a mix of vitamins A and C. They add vibrant colors and versatility to meals.

Tomatoes:
Tomatoes are rich in lycopene, a powerful antioxidant. Choose fresh tomatoes or sugar-free tomato products to avoid unnecessary added sugars.

Root Vegetables:
Sweet potatoes, carrots, and beets offer complex carbohydrates and fiber. Roasting or steaming them helps maintain their nutritional value.

Avocados:
Avocados provide healthy monounsaturated fats, fiber, and various vitamins. They contribute to satiety and help stabilize blood sugar levels.

Apples and Pears:
These fruits are high in fiber, particularly soluble fiber, which can help slow down digestion and regulate blood sugar levels.

Limit High-Glycemic Fruits:
While fruits are essential, it's advisable to
moderate high-glycemic fruits like watermelon
and pineapple to prevent rapid increases in
blood sugar.

Meal Planning:
Incorporate colorful vegetables and fruits into
every meal for a well-rounded approach.
Create salads, smoothies, and side dishes with
a mix of colorful produce.

Avoid Added Sugars:
Choose fresh, whole fruits over canned or
processed versions that may contain added
sugars.
Read labels carefully to identify and avoid
hidden sugars in packaged foods.

Portion Control:
Be mindful of portion sizes to manage overall carbohydrate intake, even from fruits and vegetables.
Pair colorful produce with lean proteins and healthy fats to create balanced meals.

By embracing a diverse array of colorful fruits and vegetables, individuals with insulin resistance can enjoy a nutrient-rich diet that supports overall health and helps manage blood sugar levels effectively.

CHAPTER SEVEN

Meal Planning Made Easy

Meal planning for an insulin resistance diet involves thoughtful consideration of food choices, portion control, and timing to help manage blood sugar levels effectively. Here's a detailed guide to make meal planning easy:

Balance Macronutrients:
Include a balance of carbohydrates, proteins, and healthy fats in each meal to promote steady blood sugar levels.
Opt for complex carbohydrates, lean proteins, and unsaturated fats.

Fiber-Rich Foods:
Prioritize high-fiber foods like whole grains, legumes, vegetables, and fruits. Fiber helps slow down digestion and regulate blood sugar.

Portion Control:
Be mindful of portion sizes to avoid overeating.
Use smaller plates to create visual cues for
appropriate serving sizes.
Distribute calories evenly across meals and
snacks throughout the day.

Frequent, Smaller Meals:
Consider eating smaller, balanced meals every
3-4 hours to prevent large fluctuations in blood
sugar levels.
Include healthy snacks between meals, such
as nuts, seeds, or veggies with hummus.

Lean Proteins:
Choose lean protein sources like poultry, fish,
tofu, legumes, and low-fat dairy to support
muscle health and satiety.

Healthy Fats:
Incorporate sources of healthy fats such as
avocados, nuts, seeds, and olive oil to add
flavor and promote a feeling of fullness.

Refined Sugar and Grain Intake: Reduce the amount of refined and processed sugar that you consume. Pick complete, unprocessed foods.

Refined grains should be avoided in favor of whole grains like quinoa, brown rice, and oats.

Meal Timing:

Aim for regular meal times to establish a consistent eating pattern.

Avoid skipping meals, as this can lead to overeating later and disrupt blood sugar levels.

Vegetables and Fruits:

Include a variety of colorful vegetables and moderate portions of fruits in your meals.

These provide essential nutrients, antioxidants, and fiber.

Meal Prepping:
Plan and prepare meals in advance to save
time and ensure healthier food choices.
Batch cook and store portions for easy access
during busy times.

Monitor Blood Sugar Levels: To learn how
different foods affect your body, check your
blood sugar levels on a regular basis.
Based on each person's response, modify your
food plan and seek advice from medical
professionals as necessary.

Consult with a Dietitian:
Seek guidance from a registered dietitian or
healthcare professional for personalized advice
tailored to your specific needs and
preferences.

Food Journaling:
Keep a food journal to track meals, snacks, and blood sugar levels. This can provide valuable insights into dietary patterns.

By incorporating these strategies into your meal planning, you can create a balanced and sustainable eating plan that supports overall health and helps manage insulin resistance effectively.

Weekly Planning Strategies

Weekly planning is a key strategy for managing an insulin resistance diet effectively. Here's a detailed guide on weekly planning strategies:

Meal Calendar:
Create a weekly meal calendar to outline your breakfast, lunch, dinner, and snacks.
Include a variety of foods to ensure a balanced intake of carbohydrates, proteins, and fats.

Grocery List: Create a thorough grocery list based on your meal plan to steer clear of impulsive unhealthy purchases.
Give lean proteins, whole grains, fresh produce, and healthy fats first priority.

Batch Cooking:
Plan a day for batch cooking and preparing meals in advance.

Cook large quantities of staples like grains, proteins, and vegetables that can be used in various dishes throughout the week.

Variety and Balance:
Ensure variety in your meals by incorporating different vegetables, proteins, and whole grains.
Balance flavors and textures to make your meals enjoyable and satisfying.

Portioning:
Portion meals into containers for easy access during the week.
This helps with portion control and ensures you have balanced options readily available.

Snack Planning:
Plan healthy snacks that align with your insulin resistance diet.
Portion snacks in advance to prevent overeating and make smart choices readily available.

Hydration Schedule:
Plan your water intake throughout the day.
Staying hydrated is crucial for overall health
and can support blood sugar management.

Weekly Shopping Routine: To guarantee you
have fresh ingredients for the week, set aside a
certain day for grocery shopping.
Adhere to your shopping list to prevent
impulsive buys.

Recipe Rotation: To keep dinners interesting,
switch up your repertoire of recipes.
To improve flavors, try varying the cooking
techniques and seasonings.

Adjust Based on Schedule:
Consider your weekly schedule when planning
meals. Opt for quick and easy recipes on busy
days.
Plan for leftovers to minimize cooking on hectic
days.

Mindful Eating:
Encourage mindful eating by creating a calm
and pleasant environment during meals.
Avoid distractions like electronic devices to
focus on enjoying your food.

Weekly Check-In:
Reflect on your insulin resistance diet progress
weekly.
Consider adjustments based on how your body
responds to different foods.

Meal Swaps:
Have alternative meal options ready in case
plans change.
Be flexible and willing to adapt your meals if
necessary.

Seek Support:
Share your meal plan with family or friends for accountability.
Encourage healthy eating habits within your household.

By incorporating these weekly planning strategies, you can establish a routine that supports your insulin resistance diet, making it easier to maintain a healthy and balanced lifestyle.

Simple Yet Effective Meal Prep Techniques

Batch Cook Proteins:
Cook a batch of lean proteins such as chicken breast, turkey, or tofu to use in various meals throughout the week.
Pre-cooked proteins make assembling balanced meals quick and convenient.

Pre-cut Vegetables:
Wash, chop, and store a variety of colorful vegetables in portioned containers.
Having pre-cut veggies readily available encourages their inclusion in meals, providing essential nutrients and fiber.

Prepare Whole Grains in Advance:
Cook whole grains like quinoa, brown rice, or barley in bulk.
Portion and store for easy access when creating balanced meals.

Make Versatile Sauces and Dressings:
Prepare healthy sauces and dressings in larger quantities and store them in separate containers.
These can add flavor to your meals without relying on high-sugar options.

Portion Control Containers:
Invest in portion control containers to pre-portion meals and snacks.
This promotes balanced eating and helps manage overall calorie intake.

Freeze Smoothie Ingredients:
Pre-pack smoothie ingredients in individual bags and freeze them.
This makes it easy to blend a nutritious smoothie quickly, combining fruits, vegetables, and protein.

Create Salad Jars:
Layer salads in mason jars, starting with dressing at the bottom and then adding sturdy ingredients.
This helps maintain freshness, and you can grab a ready-to-eat salad from the fridge.

Overnight Oats:
Prepare overnight oats by combining oats, milk, and toppings in jars.
They're a quick and healthy breakfast option that can be made in advance.

Snack Packs:
Create snack packs with a mix of nuts, seeds, and dried fruits.
This helps curb hunger between meals with a balanced and satisfying option.

Plan Theme Nights:
Designate specific nights for different types of meals, like a stir-fry night, salad night, or soup night.
Simplifies planning and ensures variety throughout the week.

Label and Date:
Label containers with the date to keep track of freshness and prevent food waste.
This ensures you prioritize consuming older meals first.

Use Slow Cooker or Instant Pot:
Utilize slow cookers or Instant Pots for easy and hands-off meal preparation.
Set it in the morning, and return to a cooked meal in the evening.

Pre-portion Healthy Snacks:
Portion out snacks like cut-up veggies, hummus, or yogurt with berries in advance. This minimizes the temptation to grab less healthy options when hunger strikes.

Stay Flexible:
While planning is key, stay flexible with your meal prep to accommodate changes in your schedule.
Having backup options ensures you stick to your insulin resistance diet even on busy days.

These simple yet effective meal prep techniques can streamline your food preparation, making it easier to stick to a balanced and insulin-friendly diet throughout the week.

CHAPTER EIGHT

Navigating Dining Out

Navigating dining out with insulin resistance requires strategic choices to maintain balanced meals and manage blood sugar levels. Here are some tips:

Check the Menu in Advance:
Review the restaurant's menu online before going to make informed choices.
Look for options with lean proteins, whole grains, and plenty of vegetables.

Choose Whole Foods:
Opt for whole, minimally processed foods instead of fried or heavily sauced dishes.
Grilled, steamed, or baked preparations are generally better choices.

Keep an Eye on Portion Sizes: Restaurant dishes are frequently larger than necessary, so keep that in mind.
Think about splitting a plate or bringing leftovers home.

Prioritize Protein: To help regulate blood sugar levels, choose foods high in protein, such as grilled chicken, fish, or tofu.
Another factor that affects feeling full is protein.

Ask for Modifications: Don't be afraid to request changes, such whole-grain alternatives or vegetable sides instead of veggie sides.
The majority of eateries are happy to fulfill specific requests.

Control Carbohydrate Intake:
Limit refined carbohydrates like white bread, pasta, and rice.
Choose whole grains or ask for substitutions when possible.

Be Mindful of Sauces and Dressings:
Many sauces and dressings can be high in added sugars.
Ask for sauces on the side or choose options with minimal added sugars.

Include Vegetables:
Ensure your meal includes a variety of colorful vegetables for added nutrients and fiber.
You can also order a side salad or steamed vegetables.

Steer Clear of Sugary Drinks: Instead of sugary drinks, choose unsweetened tea, black coffee, or water.
Blood sugar levels might surge quickly after consuming sugary beverages.

Limit Your Alcohol Consumption: If you decide to drink, make moderate drinks. Recognize that alcohol consumption can impact blood sugar levels and may necessitate modifying insulin dosage or prescription.

Mindful Eating:
Eat slowly and savor your food. This can help with portion control and digestion.
Pay attention to hunger and fullness cues.

Check Blood Sugar Levels:
Monitor your blood sugar levels before and after dining out to understand how different foods impact your body.
Adjust your insulin or medication if necessary.

Plan for Dessert:
If you want dessert, consider sharing it with others or choosing a smaller portion.
Look for options with less added sugar.

Making Informed Choices at Restaurants

Making wise decisions when dining out is crucial to successfully managing insulin resistance. Here is a guide to assist you in making better choices:

Examine the menu ahead of time:
To find healthier choices, look up the restaurant's menu online before you visit. Seek for recipes that include lots of vegetables, nutritious grains, and lean proteins.

Select Lean Proteins: Go for lean proteins like chicken, fish, or tofu that are grilled, baked, or roasted.
Steer clear of fried or breaded choices as they may include excessive levels of processed carbs and harmful fats.

Emphasize Vegetables:
Prioritize dishes with a generous serving of
vegetables.
Consider ordering a side salad or asking for
extra veggies to boost fiber content.

Control Portions:
Be mindful of portion sizes, as restaurant
servings tend to be larger than necessary.
Consider sharing a dish with a dining
companion or asking for a smaller portion.

Choose Whole Grains:
Opt for whole grains like brown rice, quinoa, or
whole wheat pasta when available.
These options provide more fiber, which can
help regulate blood sugar levels.

Be Wary of Hidden Sugars:
Watch out for hidden sugars in sauces,
dressings, and marinades.
Ask for sauces on the side or inquire about
sugar content when ordering.

Limit Refined Carbohydrates:
Minimize consumption of refined carbohydrates like white bread, white rice, and pasta. Choose whole-grain alternatives for better blood sugar control.

Request Modifications: Don't be afraid to ask for changes to your food. To suit your dietary requirements, change the sides or ask for grilled instead of fried food when placing your order.

Steer Clear of Sugary Drinks: Instead of sugary drinks, opt for unsweetened tea, black coffee, or water. Reducing added sugar consumption helps avoid sharp rises in blood sugar.

Moderate Alcohol Consumption: Use alcohol sparingly if you do. Recognize that alcohol can impact blood sugar levels, so control how much you drink.

Aim for a meal That Is Balanced: Include whole grains, veggies, and protein on your meal.
This promotes steady blood sugar levels and helps supply a variety of nutrients.

Skip or Share Desserts:
Desserts are often high in sugar and refined carbohydrates.
Consider skipping dessert or sharing a smaller portion with others.

Monitor Your Blood Sugar:
Check your blood sugar levels before and after dining out to understand how different foods affect you.
Adjust your insulin or medication as needed based on your readings.

Remain Hydrated: To stay hydrated during the meal, sip water.
It's common to confuse thirst with hunger, so staying hydrated is crucial for general health.

Social Strategies for Insulin-Friendly Eating

Social situations can present challenges when managing insulin-friendly eating, but with strategic approaches, you can navigate them successfully. Here are social strategies for insulin-friendly eating:

Communicate Dietary Preferences:
Inform friends, family, or hosts about your dietary preferences and any specific needs related to insulin resistance.
This helps create awareness and can lead to more accommodating food choices.

Suggest Insulin-Friendly Restaurants:
When planning outings, suggest restaurants that offer a variety of insulin-friendly options. Check menus in advance to ensure there are suitable choices for your dietary needs.

Lead by Example:
Demonstrate healthy eating habits to inspire
those around you.
Choose balanced options and encourage
others to make nutritious choices without
making it a focal point.

Bring a Dish:
Offer to bring a dish to social gatherings to
ensure there's something insulin-friendly
available.
This can also be an opportunity to share your
favorite healthy recipes.

Educate Friends and Family:
Share information about insulin resistance and
its dietary implications with those close to you.
This can foster understanding and support
from your social circle.

Be Assertive in Restaurants:
Don't be afraid to make specific requests or substitutions when ordering at restaurants. Most establishments are willing to accommodate dietary needs.

Portion Control:
Be mindful of portion sizes during social events.
You can enjoy the company and still make conscious choices about what and how much you eat.

Focus on Protein and Vegetables:
Prioritize protein and vegetable-based dishes when available.
These choices can help stabilize blood sugar levels and provide essential nutrients.

Remain Hydrated: To stay hydrated at social occasions, sip on water.
Additionally, it can help curb appetite and stop overindulging.

Plan Ahead for Special Occasions:
Anticipate special occasions and plan accordingly.
If you know a certain event might have limited insulin-friendly options, eat a balanced meal beforehand.

Share Your Goals:
Let your friends and family know about your health goals related to insulin resistance.
Their understanding and encouragement can positively influence your choices.

Choose Wisely at Buffets:
If faced with a buffet, survey all options before filling your plate.
Prioritize lean proteins, vegetables, and whole grains.

Practice Mindful Eating:
Be present during meals, savor each bite, and pay attention to hunger and fullness cues. This helps prevent mindless overeating in social settings.

Support System:
Surround yourself with a supportive social network that understands and respects your dietary choices.
Having a strong support system can make it easier to stick to your insulin-friendly eating plan.

Remember that balance and flexibility are key. While it's important to make informed choices, occasional indulgences are normal. Strive for consistency in insulin-friendly eating, but also allow yourself to enjoy social occasions without unnecessary stress.

CHAPTER NINE

Recipes for Success

Here's a more thorough explanation of the insulin resistance management "Recipes for Success":

Balanced Macronutrients: At each meal, aim for a proportionate amount of lean proteins, healthy fats, and complex carbohydrates. This balance offers a steady delivery of energy, which aids in blood sugar regulation.

Complex Carbohydrates: Steer clear of processed carbohydrates and toward whole grains like quinoa, brown rice, and oats. Add a lot of vegetables, as they are high in nutrients and fiber.

Lean Proteins: Choose low-fat dairy, fish, chicken, tofu, and lentils as your lean protein sources.
Protein stabilizes blood sugar levels and aids with hunger control.

Healthy Fats: Include foods like avocados, almonds, seeds, and olive oil that are high in healthy fats.
These fats can increase insulin sensitivity and promote fullness.

High-fiber diets, such as fruits, vegetables, whole grains, and legumes, should be prioritized.
Carbohydrate digestion is slowed down by fiber, which helps to avoid sharp rises in blood sugar.

Portion Control: To prevent overindulging and control calorie intake, pay attention to portion sizes.

Stabilizing blood sugar can be achieved by eating smaller, more balanced meals throughout the day.

Reduce Your Intake of Refined Carbs and Sugars: Cut Back on processed foods, sugary snacks, and drinks.

To prevent unexpected spikes in blood sugar, opt for complete, unprocessed foods.

Frequent Meals and Snacks: Try to eat at regular times, and if necessary, add nutritious snacks.

Maintaining regular eating habits can assist in keeping blood sugar levels stable.

Physical Activity:
Engage in regular aerobic exercise (e.g., brisk walking, cycling) and strength training. Exercise enhances insulin sensitivity, helping cells use glucose more effectively.

Hydration:
Stay hydrated with water and herbal teas. Proper hydration supports overall health and can aid in weight management.

Stress management: Engage in stress-relieving activities like yoga, deep breathing, or meditation. Stress management is essential since long-term stress can exacerbate insulin resistance.

Frequent Monitoring and Professional Advice: As directed by medical professionals, keep a close eye on your blood sugar levels. See a doctor or a qualified dietitian for individualized advice based on your health and needs for managing insulin resistance.

Delicious Breakfast to Start Your Day

A delicious and insulin-friendly breakfast could include:

Quinoa Breakfast Bowl:
Cooked quinoa as a base for complex carbohydrates.
Top with fresh berries for antioxidants and natural sweetness.
Add a handful of nuts or seeds for healthy fats and protein.
Finish with a dollop of Greek yogurt for added protein.

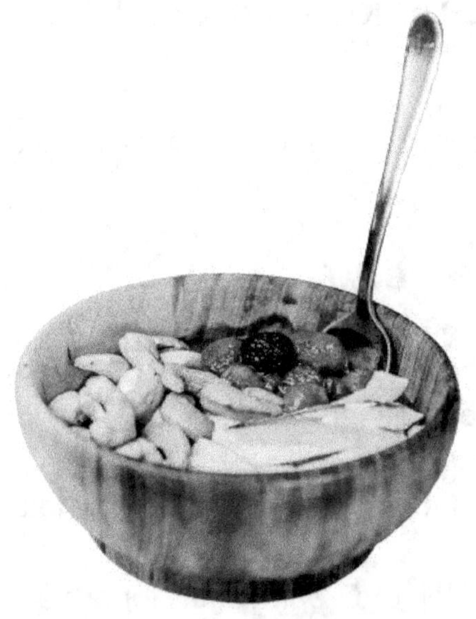

Vegetable Omelet:
Whisk together eggs and cook with a variety of colorful vegetables like spinach, bell peppers, and tomatoes.
Sprinkle some feta cheese for flavor and calcium.
Serve with a slice of whole-grain toast for additional fiber.

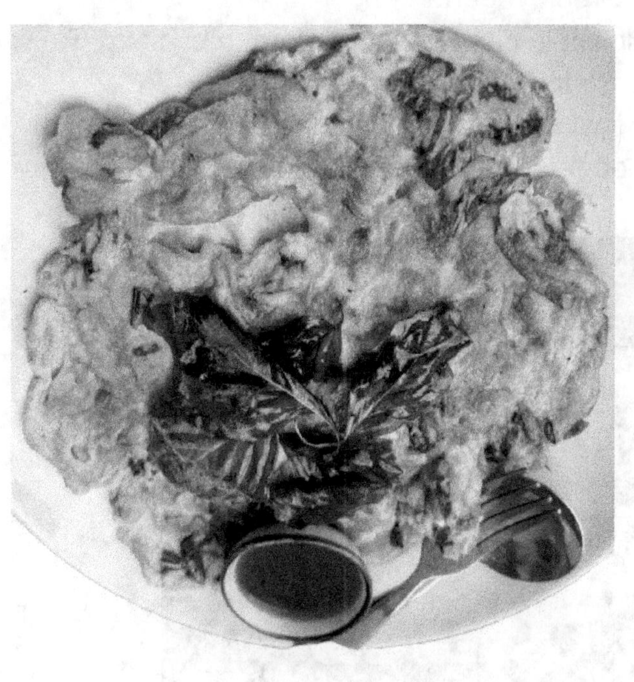

Chia Seed Pudding:

Mix chia seeds with unsweetened almond milk or Greek yogurt.

Allow it to sit overnight to form a pudding-like consistency.

Top with sliced strawberries and a sprinkle of chopped nuts for texture.

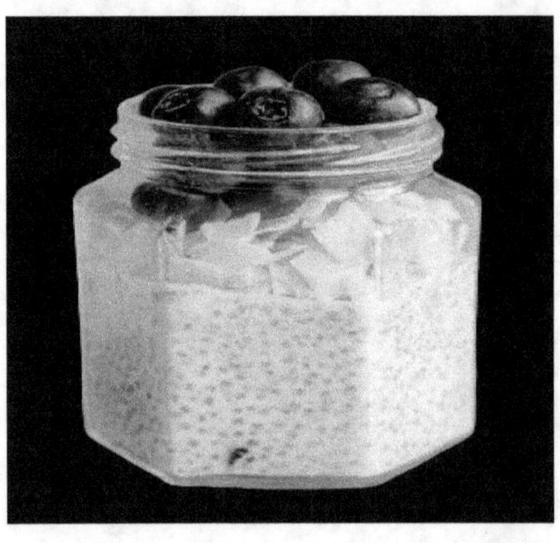

Toast with avocado and smoked salmon: For a
good source of fat, spread mashed avocado
over whole-grain bread.
Add smoked salmon on top to get your
omega-3 fatty acids.
For extra taste, add some herbs or chives.

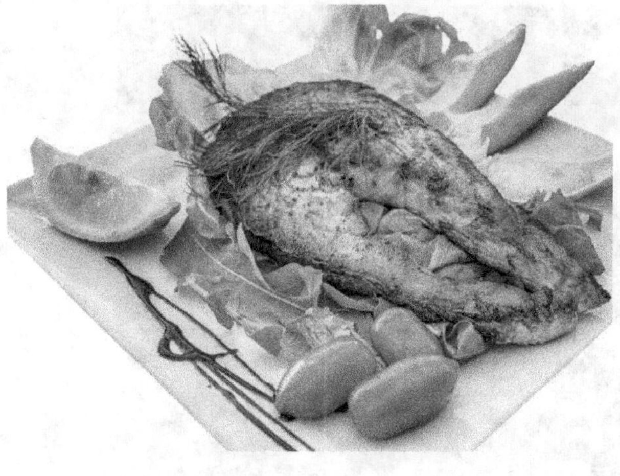

Greek Yogurt Parfait:
Layer Greek yogurt with mixed berries for a protein-packed and antioxidant-rich treat. Add a drizzle of honey or a sprinkle of cinnamon for sweetness.
Sweet Potato and Black Bean.

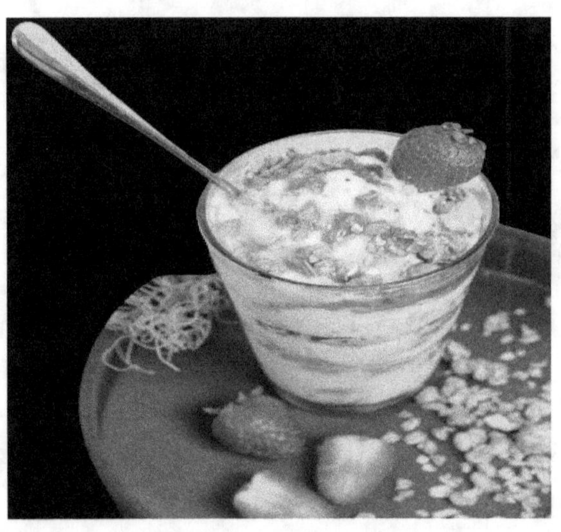

Breakfast Hash:
Sauté diced sweet potatoes, black beans, and bell peppers in olive oil.
Top with a poached or fried egg for protein and creaminess.

Remember to customize portion sizes based on your individual nutritional needs, and consider consulting with a healthcare professional or a registered dietitian for personalized advice.

Energizing Smoothie Bowls and Breakfast Ideas

Energizing smoothie bowls and breakfast ideas for insulin resistance should focus on nutrient-dense ingredients that help regulate blood sugar levels. Here are some options:

Blend spinach, kale, cucumber, and a tiny bit of green apple for sweetness in a green smoothie bowl.
For extra protein, mix with a dollop of Greek yogurt or protein powder.
Add some berries, chia seeds, and sliced almonds on top.

Berry and Avocado Smoothie Bowl:
Blend mixed berries (like blueberries and raspberries) with half an avocado for creaminess.

Include a source of protein such as cottage cheese or protein powder.
Top with granola and a sprinkle of flaxseeds for added texture.
Protein-Packed Peanut Butter

Smoothie Bowl:
Blend a banana, a tablespoon of natural peanut butter, and unsweetened almond milk.
Incorporate protein powder or Greek yogurt for added protein.
Top with sliced strawberries, a drizzle of almond butter, and crushed nuts.

Smoothie Bowl with Cocoa and Banana:
Blend almond milk, unsweetened cocoa powder, and frozen banana.
Add a dollop of Greek yogurt or a scoop of protein powder.
Add some cacao nibs and some sliced bananas on top.

Chia Seed and Almond Milk Pudding:
Mix chia seeds with unsweetened almond milk and let it sit overnight.
In the morning, top with fresh berries, a few crushed nuts, and a drizzle of honey.

Coconut and Mango Smoothie Bowl:
Blend frozen mango with coconut milk and a splash of lime juice.
Add protein with Greek yogurt or protein powder.
Top with shredded coconut, sliced mango, and a sprinkle of pumpkin seeds.

Protein-Packed Morning Delights

Protein-rich breakfast foods for insulin resistance can help control blood sugar levels and provide you energy for the entire day. Here are some suggestions:

To make egg muffins, whisk together eggs, finely chopped veggies, and cheese.
After filling muffin tins, bake until mixture is set.
These portable egg muffins are low in carbs and high in protein.

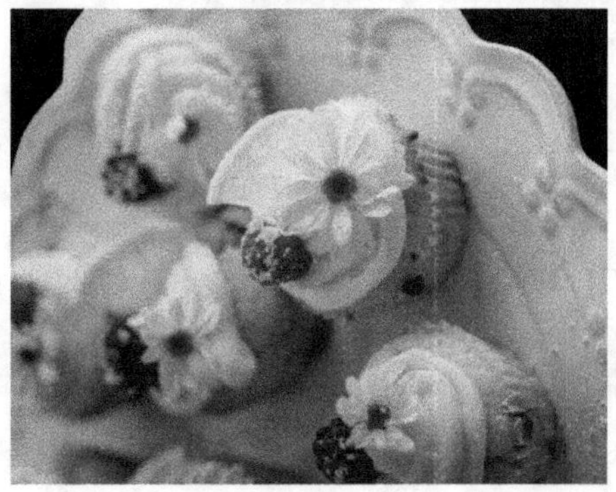

Cottage Cheese and Berries:
Mix cottage cheese with fresh berries like
strawberries or blueberries.
Cottage cheese is a good source of protein,
and the berries add natural sweetness and
fiber.

Greek Yogurt Parfait:
Layer Greek yogurt with sliced almonds, chia
seeds, and berries.
Greek yogurt is high in protein, and the
combination provides a satisfying and
nutritious breakfast.

Salmon and Cream Cheese Roll-Ups:
Spread a thin layer of cream cheese on
smoked salmon slices.
Roll them up and enjoy a protein-rich, omega-3
fatty acid-packed breakfast.

Turkey and Avocado Wrap:
Wrap sliced turkey breast and avocado in a
whole-grain tortilla.
This combination offers lean protein and
healthy fats.

Protein-Packed Smoothie:
Blend together protein powder, unsweetened
almond milk, and a handful of berries.
Optionally, add a spoonful of almond butter for
extra richness and protein.

Chia Seed Pudding with Nuts:
Make chia seed pudding with unsweetened
almond milk and top with chopped nuts.
Chia seeds are a good source of protein and
healthy fats.

Almond Flour Pancakes:
Prepare pancakes using almond flour instead
of regular flour.
Top with Greek yogurt and a few sliced
strawberries for a protein boost.

Tofu Scramble:
Sauté tofu with vegetables like spinach,
tomatoes, and bell peppers.
Season with herbs and spices for a flavorful,
plant-based protein breakfast.

Protein-Packed Oatmeal:
Cook oats with milk or a milk substitute and stir
in protein powder.
Top with nuts, seeds, or a dollop of Greek
yogurt for added protein.

CHAPTER TEN

LunchTime Favorites For Sustained Energy

Lunchtime favorites for sustained energy with a focus on managing insulin resistance should include a combination of lean proteins, fiber-rich carbohydrates, and healthy fats. Here are some ideas:

Grilled Chicken Salad:
Grill chicken breast and place it on a bed of mixed greens.
Add colorful vegetables like cherry tomatoes, cucumbers, and bell peppers.
Drizzle with olive oil and balsamic vinegar for healthy fats.

Quinoa & Veggie Bowl: Prepare the quinoa and then toss it with sautéed or roasted veggies.
Include a source of protein, like grilled tofu or chickpeas.

Add some feta cheese and a squeeze of lemon on top.

Salmon and Quinoa Wrap:
Fill a whole-grain wrap with grilled salmon, quinoa, and a mix of greens.
Include avocado slices for healthy fats.
Wrap it up for a convenient and nutritious lunch.

Turkey and Avocado Lettuce Wraps:
Use large lettuce leaves as wraps and fill them with turkey slices, avocado, and tomato.
Add a spread of hummus for extra flavor and fiber.

To make a Mediterranean Chickpea Salad, mix chickpeas with cucumber, feta cheese, cherry tomatoes, and olives.
Toss with lemon juice, olive oil, and herbs for a light and high-protein salad.

Stir-fried Tofu with Colorful veggies: Combine tofu with a range of vibrant veggies, such as bell peppers, broccoli, and snap peas.
For flavor, use homemade sauce or light soy sauce.
Serve with cauliflower or brown rice on the side.

Lentil Soup:
Prepare a hearty lentil soup with vegetables and spices.
Lentils are a good source of protein and fiber, providing lasting energy.

Sweet Potato and Black Bean Bowl:
Roast sweet potato cubes and mix with black beans, corn, and diced tomatoes.
Top with a dollop of Greek yogurt or a sprinkle of cheese.

Egg Salad Lettuce Wraps:
Make egg salad with hard-boiled eggs, Greek yogurt, and mustard.
Scoop into lettuce leaves for a low-carb, protein-rich option.

Shrimp and Vegetable Skewers:
Grill shrimp and a variety of vegetables on skewers.
Serve with quinoa or a side of roasted sweet potatoes for a balanced meal.

Wholesome Salads and Filling Sandwiches

Here are some suggestions for hearty salads and substantial sandwiches that are designed to help manage insulin resistance:

Healthy Salads:

A salad of mixed greens with grilled chicken breast and avocado.
Add pieces of avocado, cucumber, and cherry tomatoes.
For extra texture, add a drizzle of olive oil and sprinkle with seeds.

Salmon and Quinoa Salad:
Baked or grilled salmon on a base of quinoa.
Toss in spinach, cherry tomatoes, and chopped bell peppers.
Dress with a light vinaigrette or lemon-tahini dressing.

Mediterranean Chickpea Salad:

Chickpeas mixed with cherry tomatoes, cucumber, olives, and feta cheese.
Dress with olive oil, lemon juice, and a pinch of oregano.

Spinach and Berry Salad:
Fresh spinach leaves with mixed berries (strawberries, blueberries).
Add walnuts or almonds for crunch.
Dress with a balsamic vinaigrette.

Turkey and Quinoa Bowl:
Sliced turkey breast with cooked quinoa.
Mix in diced apples, celery, and a sprinkle of feta cheese.
Toss with a light citrus dressing.

Filling Sandwiches:

Grilled Chicken Wrap:
Grilled chicken strips wrapped in a whole-grain
tortilla.
Include lettuce, tomato, and a smear of
hummus or avocado.

Veggie and Hummus Sandwich:
Whole-grain bread with hummus spread.
Layer with cucumber, tomato, bell peppers,
and spinach.

Greek yogurt, celery, and a hint of mustard are
the ingredients of this tuna salad lettuce wrap
recipe.
Low-carb version: scoop into large lettuce
leaves.

Whole-grain bread stacked with tomato slices,
fresh mozzarella, and basil leaves is known as
a caprese sandwich.
Drizzle with a little olive oil and balsamic glaze.

Whole-grain bread topped with mashed
avocado and hard-boiled eggs.
Spread on whole-grain bread, then top with
tomato and lettuce.

Turkey and Cranberry Wrap:
Turkey slices with cranberry sauce wrapped in
a whole-grain tortilla.
Include spinach leaves and a smear of cream
cheese.

Grilled Vegetable Panini:
Grilled zucchini, eggplant, and bell peppers on
whole-grain bread.
Add a slice of mozzarella and press in a panini
maker.

Chicken Caesar Lettuce Wraps:
Grilled chicken strips with Caesar dressing.
Wrap in large lettuce leaves with cherry
tomatoes.

Soup Creations for Balanced Nutrition

Creating balanced and nutritious soups is a great way to support insulin resistance. Here are some ideas for soup creations:

Vegetable and Lentil Soup:
Combine a variety of colorful vegetables like carrots, celery, and bell peppers with lentils. Use vegetable broth and add herbs and spices for flavor.

Chicken and Quinoa Soup:
Cooked quinoa, shredded chicken, and an assortment of vegetables (such as spinach, carrots, and peas).
Use a low-sodium chicken broth and season with herbs like thyme and rosemary.

Tomato and Chickpea Soup:

Simmer tomatoes, chickpeas, onions, and garlic in vegetable broth.
Add a touch of olive oil and garnish with fresh basil.

Minestrone Soup:
Combine beans, whole-grain pasta, tomatoes, and an array of vegetables (zucchini, carrots, and spinach).
Season with Italian herbs and vegetable broth.

Turkey and Vegetable Chili:
Ground turkey, kidney beans, tomatoes, and bell peppers in a chili base.
Include chili powder, cumin, and paprika for flavor.

Spinach and White Bean Soup:
White beans, spinach, tomatoes, and onions cooked in vegetable broth.
Season with garlic, thyme, and a squeeze of lemon juice.

Broccoli and Cheddar Soup:

Steamed broccoli blended with low-fat cheddar cheese.
Use low-sodium vegetable or chicken broth as the base.

Asian-Inspired Tofu and Vegetable Soup:
Tofu cubes, bok choy, mushrooms, and sliced carrots in a miso or vegetable broth.
Add soy sauce, ginger, and garlic for an Asian flair.

Butternut Squash and Apple Soup:
Roasted butternut squash and apples blended with vegetable broth.
Season with cinnamon and nutmeg for sweetness.

Spicy Shrimp and Quinoa Soup:
Quinoa, shrimp, tomatoes, and bell peppers in a spicy broth.
Include cayenne pepper, paprika, and a squeeze of lime for flavor.

When creating soups, aim for a balance of lean proteins, complex carbohydrates, and healthy fats. Use herbs and spices for seasoning instead of excessive salt, and consider adding a variety of colorful vegetables for added nutrients. Adjust portion sizes to suit individual needs, and consult with healthcare professionals for personalized advice.

CHAPTER ELEVEN

Dinner Delights for Insulin Sensitivity

Dinner delights for insulin sensitivity should focus on balanced meals with a mix of lean proteins, complex carbohydrates, and healthy fats. Here are some ideas:

Grilled Salmon with Quinoa and Roasted Vegetables:
Grilled salmon for omega-3 fatty acids.
Quinoa is a complex carbohydrate and roasted vegetables for fiber and nutrients.

Turkey and Vegetable Stir-Fry:
Lean ground turkey or turkey strips stir-fried
with a variety of colorful vegetables.
Serve over cauliflower rice or brown rice for a
balanced meal.
Baked Chicken Breast with Sweet

Potato and Broccoli:
Baked chicken breast for protein.
Sweet potatoes as a complex carbohydrate
and broccoli for added fiber.

Eggplant and Chickpea Curry:
Eggplant and chickpeas simmered in a flavorful
tomato-based curry.
Serve with quinoa or whole-grain rice for
completeness.

Cauliflower and Lentil Stew:
Lentils and cauliflower in a hearty stew with a
mix of spices.
Add a side of green salad for freshness.

Zucchini Noodles with Pesto and Grilled Chicken:
Zucchini noodles topped with homemade pesto.
Grilled chicken strips for protein.

Tofu and Vegetable Skewers:
Tofu cubes and a variety of vegetables grilled on skewers.
Pair with a side of quinoa or a small portion of whole-grain couscous.

Salmon and Asparagus Foil Packets:
Salmon filet and asparagus seasoned and cooked in foil packets.
Serve with a side of quinoa or wild rice.

Spaghetti Squash with Turkey Bolognese:
Spaghetti squash strands with a lean
turkey-based Bolognese sauce.
Sprinkle with grated Parmesan for added
flavor.

Chickpea and Vegetable Curry:
Chickpeas and a mix of vegetables in a
coconut milk-based curry.
Serve over quinoa or cauliflower rice.

Always remember to monitor portion sizes,
prioritize whole, unprocessed foods, and select
cooking techniques such as baking, steaming,
or grilling.
Incorporating a range of vibrant veggies and
herbs not only enhances taste but also offers
vital nutrients. Seek guidance from medical
professionals for tailored recommendations
based on specific medical requirements.

Lean Proteins and Flavorful Vegetable Dishes

Incorporating lean proteins and flavorful vegetable dishes is a smart approach for managing insulin resistance. Here are ideas for combining these elements:

Lean Proteins:

Grilled Chicken Breast:
Season with herbs like rosemary and thyme for added flavor.
Pair with a colorful vegetable side or salad.

Turkey Patties with Herbs:
Mix ground turkey with fresh herbs like parsley and cilantro.
Grill or bake and serve with steamed vegetables.

Baked Fish with Lemon and Dill:
Choose white fish like cod or tilapia.
Bake with a drizzle of olive oil, lemon, and
fresh dill.

Tofu Stir-Fry:
Marinate tofu in a low-sodium soy sauce or a
ginger-garlic marinade.
Stir-fry with an assortment of colorful
vegetables.

Lean Beef Skewers:
Skewer lean beef cubes with bell peppers and
onions.
Grill and serve with a side of roasted Brussels
sprouts.

Egg White Omelette:
Whisk egg whites and cook with spinach,
tomatoes, and mushrooms.
Top with fresh herbs for added flavor.

Salmon Salad:
Poached or grilled salmon served on a bed of
mixed greens.
Add cherry tomatoes, cucumber, and a light
vinaigrette.

Flavorful Vegetable Dishes:

**Roasted Vegetables with Garlic and
Rosemary:**
Toss vegetables like carrots, Brussels sprouts,
and sweet potatoes in olive oil, garlic, and
rosemary.
Roast until caramelized.

Garlic and Lemon Sautéed Spinach: Finely
chop garlic and sauté fresh spinach in olive oil.
Add a squeeze of lemon juice to finish.

Curry Roasted Cauliflower:
Toss cauliflower florets in curry powder and
roast until golden.
Garnish with fresh cilantro.

Stir-Fried Broccoli with Ginger:
Stir-fry broccoli with fresh ginger, garlic, and a
splash of low-sodium soy sauce.
Top with sesame seeds.

Zucchini Noodles with Tomato Basil Sauce:
Spiralize zucchini into noodles and toss with a
homemade tomato and basil sauce.
Add grilled chicken for protein.

Balsamic Glazed Grilled Asparagus: Drizzle
balsamic glaze over grilled asparagus stalks.
For extra crunch, add chopped nuts as a
sprinkle.

Sauté spinach and mushrooms: Sauté
spinach and mushrooms in a little olive oil and
balsamic vinegar.
Add a dash of red pepper flakes, salt, and
pepper for seasoning.

Alternative Grains and Smarts Carbohydrate Choices

For an insulin resistance diet, incorporating alternative grains and smart carbohydrate choices can help manage blood sugar levels more effectively. Here are some options:

Alternative Grains:

Quinoa:
A complete protein source with a good balance of amino acids.
Rich in fiber, vitamins, and minerals.

Brown rice has more minerals and fiber than white rice.
delivers a consistent energy release.

Buckwheat: A high-fiber, high-protein grain free of gluten.
Has a high content of vital minerals and antioxidants.

Barley:
High in soluble fiber, which can help regulate
blood sugar.
Adds a chewy texture to dishes.

Farro:
Ancient grain with a nutty flavor.
Good source of protein, fiber, and vitamins.

Millet:
Gluten-free grain with a mild flavor.
Rich in nutrients, including magnesium and
phosphorus.

Smart Carbohydrate Choices:

Sweet Potatoes:
Rich in fiber, vitamins, and antioxidants.
Has a lower glycemic index compared to
regular potatoes.

Legumes (Beans, Lentils, Chickpeas):
High in fiber and protein, which helps stabilize
blood sugar.
Rich in essential nutrients and minerals.

Select pasta that is made from whole grains,
such as brown rice or whole wheat.
Greater than refined pasta in terms of nutrients
and fiber content.

Oats: Rich in soluble fiber called beta-glucans.
can enhance the sensitivity to insulin.

Berries:
Low in sugar and high in fiber, antioxidants,
and vitamins.
Blueberries, strawberries, and raspberries are
good choices.

Non-Starchy Vegetables:
Include a variety of colorful vegetables like broccoli, cauliflower, leafy greens, and bell peppers.
Low in calories and rich in fiber and nutrients.

Quinoa Pasta:
An alternative to traditional pasta made from quinoa flour.
Provides a gluten-free option with a good protein content.

Sprouted Grain Bread:
Contains sprouted grains, which may enhance nutrient absorption.
Typically lower in carbohydrates and higher in fiber.

CHAPTER TWELVE

Satisfying Snacks and Desserts

Snacks and desserts for an insulin resistance diet should focus on nutrient-dense options that provide satisfaction without causing rapid spikes in blood sugar levels. Here are some ideas:

Satisfying Snacks:

Greek Yogurt with Berries:
Choose plain, unsweetened Greek yogurt.
Top with fresh berries for natural sweetness and added antioxidants.

A handful of nuts: Choose a blend of pistachios, almonds, or walnuts.
Nuts supply protein and good fats for long-lasting energy.

Hummus-topped carrot, cucumber, and bell pepper sticks make a tasty snack.
For a satisfying blend of protein and fiber, dip in hummus.

Hard-boiled eggs are a quick and high-protein snack.
For flavor, add a dash of salt or pepper.

Whole Grain Crackers with Cheese: Serve a modest amount of cheese with whole grain crackers.
A balance of complex carbs and protein is provided by the combination.

Chia Seed Pudding: Combine unsweetened almond milk and chia seeds.
Allow it to settle until it takes on the consistency of pudding.
For extra sweetness, sprinkle some berries on top.

Cottage Cheese with Pineapple:
Choose low-fat or fat-free cottage cheese.
Add fresh pineapple chunks for a sweet and
protein-rich snack.

Avocado on Rice Cakes:
Spread mashed avocado on whole-grain rice
cakes.
Sprinkle with a pinch of salt or add cherry
tomatoes for extra flavor.

Delicious Desserts:

Dark Chocolate-Covered Almonds: Savor a
tiny serving of almonds covered in dark
chocolate.
Almonds offer good lipids, and dark chocolate
is high in antioxidants.

Apples Baked with Cinnamon: Cut apples into slices and bake them with a dash of cinnamon.
For creaminess, add a dollop of Greek yogurt on top.

Greek yogurt and mixed berries make up a berry parfait.
For crunch, add a sprinkling of nuts or seeds.

Chia Seed and Berry Sorbet:
Blend frozen berries with chia seeds.
Allow it to freeze for a refreshing and fiber-rich dessert.

Grilled Peaches with Ricotta:
Grill peach halves and top with a spoonful of ricotta cheese.
Drizzle with a touch of honey.

Bake the pear halves after dusting them with cinnamon.
Top with a spoonful of fat-free whipped cream and serve.

Yogurt and Nut Bowl: Mix plain yogurt, almonds, and honey in a bowl.
offers a filling combination of healthy fats and protein.

Quick and Nourishing Snack Recipes

Here are 15 quick and nourishing snack recipes tailored for an insulin resistance diet:

Almond Butter and Banana Slices:
Spread natural almond butter on banana slices.
Almonds provide healthy fats and protein, while bananas offer natural sweetness.

Cucumber and Hummus Bites:
Slice cucumber into rounds and top with hummus.
A refreshing and satisfying snack with a mix of fiber and protein.

Cherry Tomatoes with Mozzarella:
Pair cherry tomatoes with mozzarella cheese.
Tomatoes offer antioxidants, and mozzarella provides protein.

Edamame Bowl:
Steam edamame and sprinkle it with sea salt.
A high-protein, fiber-rich snack that satisfies
hunger.

Yogurt Parfait with Berries:
Layer plain Greek yogurt with mixed berries.
Greek yogurt adds protein, and berries provide
natural sweetness and antioxidants.

Hard-Boiled Egg and Avocado:
Slice a hard-boiled egg and top with mashed
avocado.
Eggs offer protein, while avocado contributes
healthy fats.

Trail Mix with Nuts and Seeds:
Create a mix of almonds, walnuts, pumpkin
seeds, and a few dark chocolate pieces.
A nutrient-dense combination of healthy fats
and antioxidants.

Carrot Sticks with Guacamole:
Dip carrot sticks into homemade guacamole.
Carrots offer crunch, and avocados provide
monounsaturated fats.

Whole Grain Crackers with Tuna Salad:
Top whole-grain crackers with a mix of tuna,
Greek yogurt, and diced celery.
A protein-rich and satisfying snack.

**Apple Slices with Almond Butter and
Cinnamon:**
Spread almond butter on apple slices.
Sprinkle it with cinnamon for added flavor.

Roasted Chickpeas: Combine your preferred
spices and olive oil with the chickpeas.
Roast till crispy for a satisfyingly crunchy,
high-protein snack.

Celery Sticks with Peanut Butter:
Fill celery sticks with natural peanut butter.
A classic combination of crunch and
creaminess.

Greek Yogurt and Granola Parfait:
Layer Greek yogurt with a small amount of
granola.
Choose a granola with lower added sugars for
a balanced snack.

Cheese and Whole Wheat Pita: Combine
slices of whole wheat pita with cheese cubes.
gives a combination of complex carbs and
protein.

fruit and Cottage Cheese Bowl: Mix together
cottage cheese and various fruits.

Guilt-Free Desserts for Sweet Cravings

Guilt-free desserts for sweet cravings on an insulin resistance diet prioritize whole, minimally processed ingredients and limit added sugars. Here are some ideas:

Dark Chocolate-Covered Strawberries:
Dip fresh strawberries in melted dark chocolate.
Dark chocolate contains antioxidants and is lower in sugar than milk chocolate.

Baked Apple with Cinnamon:
Slice apples and bake with a sprinkle of cinnamon.
Cinnamon adds flavor without the need for additional sugar.

Chia Seed Pudding:
Mix chia seeds with unsweetened almond milk and let it thicken.
Top with a few berries or a small amount of unsweetened coconut.

Greek Yogurt with Honey and Nuts:
Choose plain Greek yogurt and drizzle with a touch of honey.
Add a sprinkle of chopped nuts for crunch.

Homemade Fruit Sorbet:
Blend frozen berries or mango chunks with a splash of water.
No added sugars, just the natural sweetness of the fruit.

Avocado Chocolate Mousse:
Blend ripe avocado with unsweetened cocoa
powder and a touch of honey.
Provides a creamy, chocolatey dessert rich in
healthy fats.

Baked Pears with Cinnamon and Walnuts:
Bake pear halves with a sprinkle of cinnamon
and chopped walnuts.
A warm, comforting dessert without added
sugars.

Coconut and Almond Energy Balls:
Mix shredded coconut, almond flour, and a
touch of almond butter.
Form into small balls for a satisfying and
energy-boosting treat.

Yogurt Berry Parfait:
Layer plain Greek yogurt with fresh berries.
Add a sprinkle of nuts or seeds for texture.

Pumpkin Spice Chia Pudding:
Combine chia seeds with pumpkin puree and a dash of pumpkin spice.
Sweeten with a touch of maple syrup or a sugar substitute.

Cocoa-Dusted Almonds:
Toss almonds in unsweetened cocoa powder.
Provides a chocolatey flavor without excess sugar.

Baked Peach with Cinnamon:
Halve peaches, sprinkle with cinnamon, and bake until tender.
Enjoy the natural sweetness of baked fruit.

Raspberry Coconut Bliss Balls:
Blend raspberries with shredded coconut and almond flour.
Roll into bite-sized balls for a fruity, coconut treat.

Berry and Mint Infused Water:
Infuse water with fresh berries and a few mint
leaves.
A refreshing, sugar-free alternative to sugary
beverages.

These guilt-free desserts focus on natural
sweetness from fruits, minimal added sugars,
and the use of wholesome ingredients. Portion
control remains important, and these treats can
be enjoyed as part of a balanced diet for
individuals managing insulin resistance.
Always consult with healthcare professionals or
a registered dietitian for personalized dietary
advice.

CHAPTER THIRTEEN

Lifestyle Strategies for Long-Term Success

Lifestyle strategies for long-term success in managing insulin resistance involve adopting sustainable habits that promote overall health. Here are key strategies:

Balanced and Nutrient-Dense Diet:
Prioritize whole, unprocessed foods, including lean proteins, whole grains, colorful vegetables, and healthy fats.
Monitor portion sizes and choose foods with a low glycemic index to help regulate blood sugar levels.

Frequent Exercise: Take part in regular physical activity, which should include strength training as well as cardio exercises like cycling, jogging, or walking.
Try to get in at least 150 minutes a week of moderate-to-intense activity.

Weight management is the practice of either maintaining or striving for a healthy weight. Reducing excess weight can lower the risk of problems linked to insulin resistance and increase insulin sensitivity.

Hydration: Throughout the day, sip water to be properly hydrated.
Choose water, herbal teas, or other low-calorie drinks instead of sugar-filled ones.

Consistent Meal Timing:
Establish regular meal times to help regulate blood sugar levels.
Avoid long periods between meals to prevent sharp spikes and crashes in blood glucose.

Eat with awareness: Develop mindful eating by being aware of your body's signals of hunger and fullness.
For improved digestion and satisfaction, chew meals well and enjoy the tastes.

Sufficient Sleep: Aim for seven to nine hours of sound sleep every night.
Sleep is crucial for general health because it might have a detrimental impact on insulin sensitivity.

Stress management: Include stress-relieving exercises like yoga, deep breathing, meditation, or mindfulness.
Stress management is essential since long-term stress can exacerbate insulin resistance.

Education and Support:
Stay informed about insulin resistance and its management through reliable sources.
Seek support from healthcare professionals, dietitians, or support groups to stay motivated and on track.

Consistent Lifestyle Changes:
Focus on making gradual, sustainable lifestyle changes.
Avoid extreme diets or restrictive practices, as they may not be maintainable in the long term.

Regular Health Screenings:
Attend routine health screenings, including blood pressure checks, cholesterol tests, and other relevant assessments.
Early detection and management of related conditions can contribute to long-term well-being.

Personalized Approach:
Work with healthcare professionals, including a registered dietitian, to tailor dietary and lifestyle recommendations to individual needs

Understand that what suits one individual might not suit another.
Long-term management of insulin resistance requires patience, consistency, and a holistic approach. Over time, people can enhance their general health and lower their chance of developing issues related to insulin resistance by implementing these lifestyle recommendations.

Incorporating Exercise for Insulin Sensitivity

Incorporating exercise is a crucial component of managing insulin sensitivity. Regular physical activity helps the body use insulin more effectively, improving blood sugar control. Here's how you can incorporate exercise for insulin sensitivity:

Aerobic Exercise: Take part in cardiovascular or aerobic workouts including cycling, jogging, swimming, or dancing.
Try to get in at least 150 minutes a week of aerobic activity at a moderate level.

Incorporate high-intensity interval training (HIIT) into your workouts. HIIT entails brief bursts of intense activity interspersed with rest or lower-intensity sessions.
It has been demonstrated that HIIT efficiently and quickly increases insulin sensitivity.

Strength Training: Make sure to do strength training activities two days a week, minimum. Use resistance activities, such as bodyweight exercises, resistance band workouts, or weightlifting, to concentrate on your main muscle groups.

Flexibility and Balance Exercises:
Include flexibility and balance exercises such as yoga or Pilates.
These activities can complement aerobic and strength training, promoting overall fitness.

Consistency is Key:
Establish a regular exercise routine and aim for consistency.
Regularity in physical activity is important for maintaining and improving insulin sensitivity over time.

Gradual Progression: If you're new to fitness, start with low- to moderate-intensity exercises. As your fitness level rises, gradually increase the length and intensity of your workouts.

Mix Different Types of Exercise:
Combine different types of exercise to ensure a well-rounded fitness routine.
This may include a mix of aerobic, strength, and flexibility exercises throughout the week.

Post-Meal Walking:
Take short walks after meals, especially after dinner.
This can aid in glucose control and improve insulin sensitivity, particularly for those with insulin resistance.

Choose Enjoyable Activities:
Opt for physical activities you enjoy to increase
adherence to your exercise routine.
Whether it's cycling, dancing, or playing a
sport, finding enjoyable activities makes it
easier to stay active.

Monitor Blood Sugar Levels:
Monitor your blood sugar levels before and
after exercise, especially if you're taking
medication for diabetes.
This helps you understand how your body
responds to different activities.

Hydration and Recovery:
Stay hydrated during and after exercise.
Allow time for proper recovery, including
stretching and cool-down activities.

Pair Exercise with a Balanced Diet:
Combine regular exercise with a balanced, insulin-friendly diet.
The synergy between diet and physical activity is crucial for managing insulin sensitivity effectively.

Remember, it's important to tailor your exercise routine to your individual preferences, fitness level, and any underlying health conditions. Consistency over time is key to reaping the benefits of improved insulin sensitivity and overall health. Always seek guidance from healthcare professionals or fitness experts for a personalized approach.

Exercise Tips for Beginners

Starting an exercise routine as a beginner on an insulin resistance diet requires a gradual and personalized approach. Here are some exercise tips to help beginners get started:

Consult with Healthcare Professionals:
Before beginning any exercise program, consult with your healthcare team, especially if you have underlying health conditions.
Get clearance and guidance tailored to your individual health status.

Start Slow and Gradual:
Begin with low to moderate-intensity activities. For example, start with a brisk walk or gentle cycling for short durations.

Set Realistic Goals:
Establish realistic and achievable fitness goals.
Focus on building consistency rather than
pushing yourself too hard initially.

Choose Enjoyable Activities:
Pick exercises that you enjoy to increase
motivation.
This might include dancing, swimming,
gardening, or any other activity that keeps you
moving.

Include Aerobic Exercise:
Incorporate aerobic exercises like walking,
cycling, or swimming.
Aim for at least 30 minutes most days of the
week, gradually increasing duration as you
become more comfortable.

Strength Training Basics:
Include basic strength training exercises using
bodyweight or light resistance.
Focus on major muscle groups with exercises
like bodyweight squats, lunges, or wall
push-ups.

Balance and Flexibility:
Incorporate balance and flexibility exercises to
improve overall mobility.
Simple stretches or beginner-friendly yoga
poses can be beneficial.

Integrate Exercise into Daily Routine:
Look for opportunities to be active throughout
the day.
Take the stairs, park farther away, or
incorporate short walks after meals.

Hydrate and Dress Comfortably:
Stay hydrated before, during, and after
exercise.
Wear comfortable clothing and supportive
footwear to enhance your workout experience.

Consider Group Classes or Support:
Join group exercise classes or find a workout
buddy for motivation.
Classes can provide structure and social
support.

Set a Consistent Schedule:
Establish a regular exercise schedule that fits
into your routine.
Consistency is key to building a sustainable
exercise habit.

Celebrate Small Achievements:
Acknowledge and celebrate small
achievements and improvements.
This can help maintain motivation and
positivity.

Track Progress:
Keep a log of your activities and progress. This can be a helpful tool for staying accountable and adjusting your routine as needed.

Remember, the goal is to gradually build up your fitness level and make exercise a regular part of your lifestyle. Be patient with yourself, and don't be afraid to ask for guidance from healthcare professionals or fitness experts. Always prioritize safety and enjoyment in your fitness journey.

CHAPTER FOURTEEN

Stress Management Techniques

Effective stress management is crucial for individuals on an insulin resistance diet, as stress can impact blood sugar levels. Here are stress management techniques that can be beneficial:

Deep Breathing and Relaxation: To soothe the nervous system, engage in deep breathing exercises.
Another technique for calming the body and mind is progressive muscle relaxation or guided visualization.

Practice mindfulness meditation to help you
stay focused on the here and now.
Relaxation techniques like body scan
meditations and mindful breathing can help.

Yoga:
incorporate yoga into your routine, which
combines physical postures with mindfulness
and breath awareness.
Choose gentle or restorative yoga styles for
stress relief.

Regular Physical Activity:
Exercise can be an effective stress reliever.
Engage in activities you enjoy, whether it's
walking, jogging, swimming, or dancing.

Journaling:
Keep a stress journal to identify and
understand stress triggers.
Write down your thoughts and emotions,
exploring ways to manage stressors.

Social Support: Preserve close relationships with friends and family.
Express your thoughts and worries, and ask for help when you need it.

Time Management:
Organize your time efficiently to reduce feelings of overwhelm.
Prioritize tasks and break them into manageable steps.

Limit Caffeine and Stimulants:
Reduce the intake of caffeine and stimulants, which can exacerbate stress.
Opt for herbal teas or decaffeinated options.

Enough Sleep: Make sure you get a sufficient amount of good sleep every night.
Create a comfortable sleeping environment and establish a calming nighttime habit.

Healthy Nutrition: To promote general wellbeing, keep a diet that is both balanced and nutrient-rich.
Add meals high in nutrients and antioxidants that help you cope with stress.

Positive Affirmations:
Use positive affirmations to shift your mindset and focus on optimistic thoughts.
Repeat affirmations that promote self-confidence and resilience.

Hobbies & Creative Outlets: As a way to express yourself, take part in the things you enjoy doing.
Activities that involve creativity, art, or hobbies can be relieving and a way to decompress.

Technology Breaks: To lessen mental exhaustion, take breaks from screens and other electronics.
Periodically cutting off can assist reduce the stress that comes with continuous connectivity.

Nature Exposure:
Spend time outdoors and connect with nature. Walking in nature or simply being in green spaces can have a calming effect.

Professional Support:
Seek guidance from mental health professionals, such as counselors or therapists.
They can provide strategies tailored to your specific stressors.

Mindful Practices for Stress Reduction

Mindful practices can be effective for stress reduction in individuals managing insulin resistance. Here are mindful techniques that can be beneficial:

Breathe mindfully: Concentrate on your breathing, noticing each inhalation and exhalation.
Breathe deeply and deliberately to help relax the nervous system.

Body Scan Meditation:
Conduct a body scan, bringing awareness to each part of your body.
Release tension and promote relaxation by consciously relaxing each muscle group.

Eating with awareness: Take in the flavors and textures of your food.
Chew carefully; enjoy every bite; pay attention to your body's signals of hunger and fullness.

Guided Imagery:
Close your eyes and visualize a peaceful and calming scene.
Imagine the sights, sounds, and sensations to create a mental escape.

Mindful Walking:
Practice walking meditation by paying attention to each step.
Feel the sensations in your feet and notice the rhythm of your movement.

Mindful Observation:
Engage in mindful observation of your surroundings.
Focus on the details of an object, like colors, shapes, and textures.

Journal mindfully: Express your ideas and emotions in writing, free from criticism. Consider the good things in life and show thankfulness.

Kindness and Love Practice meditation to develop kindness and compassion for both yourself and other people.
To promote cheerful feelings, say affirmations like "May I be happy, may I be healthy" repeatedly.

Mindful Yoga:
Practice yoga with a focus on breath and present-moment awareness.
Connect movement with breath for a mindful and calming practice.

Mindful Listening:
Practice active listening in conversations.
Pay full attention to the speaker without formulating a response in your mind.

Use Technology Mindfully: Use it with awareness, avoiding pointless scrolling. Take breaks from your screens to clear your mind.

Mindful Pause:
Introduce mindful pauses throughout the day. Take a moment to breathe and center yourself before transitioning to the next task.

Mindful Acceptance:
Embrace acceptance of the present moment without judgment. Acknowledge thoughts and emotions without getting entangled in them.

Mindful Gratitude: Make an effort to be grateful by concentrating on your life's blessings. Express gratitude for small things on a regular basis.

Reflecting Mindfully: Allocate time for introspection.
Think about your feelings, reactions, and experiences without passing judgment.

You can develop a stronger sense of awareness and lessen the stress that comes with treating insulin resistance by implementing these mindful activities into your everyday routine. Finding the routines that you enjoy will help you stay well in the long run. Consistency is essential. Seek advice and support from healthcare specialists for individualized advice at all times.

The Impact of Stress on Insulin Resistance

Stress can have a significant impact on insulin resistance, creating a complex interplay between the body's stress response and glucose regulation. Here's how stress can influence insulin resistance:

Hormonal Response: Stress causes the release of adrenaline and cortisol, among other stress hormones.
Blood sugar levels may rise in response to elevated cortisol levels, which are part of the body's "fight or flight" reaction.

Release of Glucose: The liver releases glucose into the bloodstream in response to cortisol.
While this gives the body extra energy in stressful conditions, it can also raise blood sugar levels.

Insulin Resistance Development:
Chronic stress and consistently high levels of
cortisol may contribute to the development of
insulin resistance.
Over time, the cells become less responsive to
insulin, making it challenging for glucose to
enter cells for energy.

Stress and Abdominal Fat Accumulation:
Stress is linked to the buildup of abdominal fat.
Visceral fat in particular is associated with
insulin resistance and a higher risk of
metabolic diseases.

Unhealthy Coping Mechanisms:
Individuals under stress may adopt unhealthy
coping mechanisms, such as emotional eating
or increased consumption of sugary and
high-calorie foods.
Poor dietary choices can exacerbate insulin
resistance.

Disrupted Eating Patterns:
Stress can disrupt eating patterns, leading to irregular meal times or skipped meals. Inconsistent eating patterns can impact blood sugar levels and insulin sensitivity.

Impact on Physical Activity:
Chronic stress may contribute to a sedentary lifestyle and reduced physical activity. Lack of exercise can negatively affect insulin sensitivity.

Sleep Disruptions:
Stress often leads to sleep disturbances. Inadequate or poor-quality sleep is associated with insulin resistance and an increased risk of type 2 diabetes.

Inflammation: The body may experience inflammation as a result of ongoing stress. Insulin resistance is associated with inflammation, which may also worsen glucose metabolism.

Sympathetic Nervous System Activation: The activation of the sympathetic nervous system, part of the body's stress response, can impact insulin sensitivity. Prolonged sympathetic activation may contribute to insulin resistance.

Psychological Factors: Stress can lead to emotional and psychological factors like anxiety and depression. Mental health conditions are associated with an increased risk of insulin resistance.

Understanding and managing stress is crucial for individuals dealing with insulin resistance. Adopting stress management techniques, such as mindfulness, relaxation exercises, regular physical activity, and healthy coping mechanisms, can help mitigate the impact of stress on insulin sensitivity. It's essential to address stress as part of a comprehensive approach to overall health and well-being. Individuals should consult with healthcare professionals for personalized guidance based on their specific health conditions.

CONCLUSION

In conclusion, embracing a well-curated insulin resistance diet is not merely a dietary choice but a lifestyle commitment that fosters health and well-being. The journey toward managing insulin resistance involves making informed and mindful decisions about the foods we consume. The recipes provided in this cookbook serve as a guide, offering a diverse array of nutritious, balanced, and delicious options tailored to support stable blood sugar levels.

From energizing breakfast ideas to satisfying snacks, wholesome salads, and nourishing dinners, each recipe has been crafted to align with the principles of an insulin resistance-friendly diet.

The inclusion of lean proteins, healthy fats, and smart carbohydrate choices underscores the importance of maintaining a balanced macronutrient profile in every meal. These recipes not only cater to nutritional needs but also cater to the palate, proving that a health-conscious diet can be both enjoyable and sustainable.

Moreover, the cookbook emphasizes the significance of lifestyle factors in managing insulin resistance. Exercise tips for beginners, stress management techniques, and mindful practices are integrated to promote a holistic approach to health. Recognizing the impact of stress on insulin resistance underscores the interconnected nature of physical and mental well-being, urging individuals to adopt strategies that enhance both aspects of their health.

In essence, this insulin resistance diet cookbook is a comprehensive tool that goes beyond the confines of traditional recipe collections. It serves as a practical guide, empowering individuals to take charge of their health through mindful dietary choices, regular physical activity, and stress management. By incorporating these principles into their daily lives, individuals can embark on a journey toward improved insulin sensitivity, overall health, and long-term well-being. As with any dietary or lifestyle changes, it is advised to consult with healthcare professionals or registered dietitians for personalized guidance and support on managing insulin resistance.

Thank you for embarking on this transformative journey with our Insulin Resistance Diet Cookbook for Beginners. Your commitment to exploring a healthier and more mindful way of eating is commendable. By delving into these pages, you've taken a significant step toward understanding and managing insulin resistance through delicious, nourishing recipes.

We believe that every meal is an opportunity to support your well-being, and your decision to invest in this cookbook reflects your dedication to a healthier you. As you explore the diverse and flavorful recipes curated with your insulin resistance in mind, we hope you find joy, satisfaction, and a renewed sense of vitality in each bite.

Remember, this cookbook is more than a collection of recipes; it's a companion on your journey to better health. Your body deserves the best, and we're honored to be part of your pursuit of well-being.

Here's to a future filled with delicious, insulin-friendly meals and a healthier, happier you. Thank you for choosing our Insulin Resistance Diet Cookbook for Beginners – a stepping stone toward a life of vitality and balance.